'In this book, Maurice Apprey, a psychoanalyst for children, adolescents, and adults, describes how individuals have identifications with damaged parts of internalized images of parents and illustrates how individuals as well as ethnic, national, religious, and ideological groups are unwittingly possessed by historical events involving their ancestors. I consider Maurice Apprey one of the most integrative thinkers for creating more knowledge about the concepts of trauma, the psychology of historical events and transgenerational haunting. This important book illustrates and teaches us more about the necessity and importance of psychoanalytic study of psychical transfer in transgenerational haunting.'

Vamık Volkan, *Professor Emeritus of Psychiatry, University of Virginia; President Emeritus of International Dialogue Initiative; and past President of the Virginia Psychoanalytic Society, Turkish-American Neuropsychiatric Society, International Society of Political Psychology, and American College of Psychoanalysts*

'In this book, Apprey, a pioneer in the study of psychic phenomena expressing transgenerational transmissions of aggressivity, brilliantly shows the implications of such transmissibility for psychoanalytic theory and therapy. Taking Freud's instinct theory and reworking it into an object relations theory that can account for the temporality of psychic messaging, Apprey offers various strategies for conceptualizing how humans enact and make sense of history. Yet, of Apprey's *dramatis personae*, Freud is not the central character. Nor are the philosophers Husserl, Heidegger, Merleau-Ponty, Jean-Luc Marion, Claude Romano, et alia—all of whom Apprey mobilizes with total perspicacity. The main figure turns out to be Auden, whose celebrated 1937 poem "On This Island" prompted Apprey to think through the seeming contradictions embedded in the poetic phrase: Under what conditions are errands *voluntary*? And, if errands are truly *urgent*, then what room is left for choice, the spontaneous? Auden's "errands" would orient Apprey, like the diverging ships in the poem, sending him on a multiplex psychoanalytic errand of his own.'

Michael Uebel, *a scholar who has taught literature, literary history, and cultural theory at the University of Virginia, Georgetown University, and University of Kentucky and clinical social work at the University of Texas, Austin*

Transgenerational Haunting in Psychoanalysis

In this book, Maurice Apprey continues his unique work on transgenerational haunting to explore how events in our ancestors' lives may be renegotiated and re-subjectivized in the present from within the therapeutic dyad.

With an informed and impassioned voice that evokes the tragic psychic consequences of the unresolved, silenced tragedies and transgressions that haunt subsequent generations, Apprey illustrates how the analyst can unfold a patient's transference wishes and emancipate them from the unconscious projects, or errands, they have inherited. This can happen through a threefold process of excavating the unconscious sedimentations of ancestral history, appropriating and reactivating the ancestral errands within the transference, and subsequently decoding the patient's transference pressures. Expanding on Apprey's work about the analyst's field of inquiry and ways of listening in clinical practice, this book illuminates the potential for a resolution, rather than a re-enactment, of the traumas that can haunt a family system across generations.

Attending to the manifestation of transgenerational trauma through varied clinical material, and informed by the thinking of Sigmund Freud, among others, this book will be essential reading for all psychoanalysts and psychotherapists.

Maurice Apprey, PhD, Professor of Psychiatry Emeritus at the University of Virginia School of Medicine, trained in child and adolescent psychoanalysis at the Anna Freud Centre, London, and in adult psychoanalysis at the Institute of the Contemporary Freudian Society. He is a training and supervising psychoanalyst of the International Psychoanalytic Association.

William F. Cornell, M.A., TSTA (P), maintains an independent private practice of psychotherapy and consultation in Pittsburgh, Pennsylvania. He is the author and editor of numerous books in transactional analysis and psychoanalysis. A co-editor of the *Transactional Analysis Journal* for 15 years, he is now the editor of the Routledge book series "Innovations in Transactional Analysis." He is a recipient of the Eric Berne Memorial Award and the European Association for Transactional Analysis Gold Medal in recognition of his writing.

Relational Perspectives Book Series

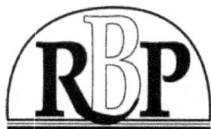

R̶B̶P̶

The Relational Perspectives Book Series (RPBS) publishes books that grow out of or contribute to the relational tradition in contemporary psychoanalysis. The term *relational psychoanalysis* was first used by Greenberg and Mitchell[1] to bridge the traditions of interpersonal relations, as developed within interpersonal psychoanalysis and object relations, as developed within contemporary British theory. But, under the seminal work of the late Stephen A. Mitchell, the term *relational psychoanalysis* grew and began to accrue to itself many other influences and developments. Various tributaries—interpersonal psychoanalysis, object relations theory, self psychology, empirical infancy research, feminism, queer theory, sociocultural studies and elements of contemporary Freudian and Kleinian thought—flow into this tradition, which understands relational configurations between self and others, both real and fantasied, as the primary subject of psychoanalytic investigation.

We refer to the relational tradition, rather than to a relational school, to highlight that we are identifying a trend, a tendency within contemporary psychoanalysis, not a more formally organized or coherent school or system of beliefs. Our use of the term *relational* signifies a dimension of theory and practice that has become salient across the wide spectrum of contemporary psychoanalysis. Now under the editorial supervision of Adrienne Harris and Eyal Rozmarin, the Relational Perspectives Book Series originated in 1990 under the editorial eye of the late Stephen A. Mitchell. Mitchell was the most prolific and influential of the originators of the relational tradition. Committed to dialogue among psychoanalysts, he abhorred the authoritarianism that dictated adherence to a rigid set of beliefs or technical restrictions. He championed open discussion, comparative and integrative approaches, and promoted new voices across the generations. Mitchell was later joined by the late Lewis Aron, also a visionary and influential writer, teacher and leading thinker in relational psychoanalysis.

Included in the Relational Perspectives Book Series are authors and works that come from within the relational tradition, those that extend and develop that tradition, and works that critique relational approaches or compare and contrast them with alternative points of view. The series includes our most distinguished senior psychoanalysts, along with younger contributors who bring fresh vision. Our aim is to enable a deepening of relational thinking while reaching across disciplinary and social boundaries in order to foster an inclusive and international literature.

A full list of titles in this series is available at www.routledge.com/Relational-Perspectives-Book-Series/book-series/LEARPBS.

Note

1 Greenberg, J. & Mitchell, S. (1983). *Object Relations in Psychoanalytic Theory.* Cambridge, MA: Harvard University Press.

Transgenerational Haunting in Psychoanalysis

Toxic Errands

Maurice Apprey

Edited by
William F. Cornell
With contributions
by Edward T. Novak

Routledge
Taylor & Francis Group

LONDON AND NEW YORK

Designed cover image: © Getty Images

First published 2024
by Routledge
4 Park Square, Milton Park, Abingdon, Oxon OX14 4RN

and by Routledge
605 Third Avenue, New York, NY 10158

Routledge is an imprint of the Taylor & Francis Group, an informa business

British Library Cataloguing-in-Publication Data
A catalogue record for this book is available from the British Library

This book contains material of a highly sensitive nature including
descriptions of child sexual abuse.

ISBN: 978-1-032-48429-7 (hbk)
ISBN: 978-1-032-48430-3 (pbk)
ISBN: 978-1-003-38902-6 (ebk)

DOI: 10.4324/9781003389026

Typeset in Times New Roman
by Apex CoVantage, LLC

For
Barkers, Sarah, Thelma, Laud, and Swayzine,
Three generations of ancestors
who continue to till the fertile fields of reference to
my inner world.

Contents

Acknowledgments

Editor's Introduction: Portions of this book have been previously published in a different form in *Self-Examination in Psychoanalysis and Psychotherapy: Countertransference and Subjectivity in Clinical Practice*, William F. Cornell, 2019, Routledge.

Chapter 2: "Urgent Voluntary Errands": W.H. Auden and my very first intuitive grasp of psychoanalysis. This chapter was first published in 2016 as the lead article for the inaugural but erstwhile *ejournal of the International Psychoanalytic Association*.

Chapter 3: Apprey, M. (2003). "Repairing History: Reworking Transgenerational Trauma" (pp. 3–27) in: Moss, D. (ed.) *Hating in the First Person Plural*. Other Press. Reprinted with permission.

Chapter 4: Maurice Apprey Interviewed by William F. Cornell (2019), "Scripting" Inhabitations of Unwelcome Guests, Hosts, and Ghosts: Unpacking Elements That Constitute Transgenerational Haunting, *Transactional Analysis Journal*, 49:4, 339–351, DOI: 10.1080/03621537.2019.1650234 © International Transactional Analysis Association, reprinted by permission of Taylor & Francis Ltd, www.tandfonline.com, on behalf of International Transactional Analysis Association.

Chapter 5: Representing, Theorizing and Reconfiguring the Concept of Transgenerational Haunting in Order to Facilitate Healing. This was the lead chapter in *Trans-Generational Trauma and the Other: Dialogues across History and Difference*. Edited by Sue Grand and Jill Salberg in 2017, reprinted by permission of the publisher (Taylor & Francis Ltd, www.tandfonline.com).

Chapter 6: Apprey, M. "Difference and The Awakening of Wounds in Intercultural Psychoanalysis," *The Psychoanalytic Quarterly*, (2006) 75:1, reprinted by permission of the publisher (Taylor & Francis Ltd, www.tandfonline.com).

Chapter 8: Apprey, M. "A Pluperfect Errand: A Turbulent Return to Beginnings in the Transgenerational Transmission of Destructive Aggression," *Free Associations: Psychoanalysis and Culture, Media, Groups, Politics* (2014), is here reprinted with permission.

Chapter 9: Three Leitmotifs for Sequencing and Transforming the Process of Transgenerational Transmission of Destructive Aggression. This chapter was a contribution to the *Psychohistory Forum* in 2022.

Chapter 11: Apprey, M. "'Containing the Uncontainable': The Return of the Phantom and Its Reconfiguration in Ethnonational Conflict Resolution", *The American Journal of Psychoanalysis* (2014), © 2014, Springer Nature. Reprinted with permission.

Chapter 13: Emancipation from Institutionalization: A Case Study on Transgenerational Hauntings. Edward T. Novak. This chapter was originally published in *The Transactional Analysis Journal* in 2022. It is published here with the permission of Routledge.

Chapter 14: *THROWN:* A Personal Narrative of Psychoanalysis and Toxic Errands. William F. Cornell. Portions of this chapter were previously published in a different form in *Intimacies: A New World of Relational Life*. A. Frank, P.T. Clough, & S. Seidman, Eds., 2013, Routledge.

About the Author, Editor, and Contributors

Maurice Apprey, PhD, is Professor of Psychiatry Emeritus at the University of Virginia School of Medicine, where he taught psychoanalytic thought to residents of psychiatry and psychology, medical students, and hospital chaplains for over 40 years. A non-medical psychoanalyst, he was a member of the Academy of Distinguished Educators who teamed up with physicians to teach interviewing skills and other clinical competencies to first-year medical students. He trained in child and adolescent psychoanalysis at the Hampstead Clinic, now the Anna Freud Centre, London, and in adult psychoanalysis at the New York Freudian Society, now the Institute of the Contemporary Freudian Society, where he also served a teaching, training, and supervising psychoanalyst. In addition, he served as a teaching and supervising psychoanalyst for PSIKE, an IPA training institute in Istanbul, for 16 years. A student of Amedeo Giorgi, an American phenomenological psychological researcher and of psychoanalysis, he keeps the tension between description and interpretation alive in order to be faithful to the mind of a subject without seeking premature closure or getting ahead of the patient.

Apprey is interested in the transformation of mental structures in psychoanalysis going back generations, if and when he can. Outside psychoanalysis, he has served as a dean of African American affairs and an associate vice-president of student affairs at the University of Virginia, where he created academic advancement programs for underserved and disadvantaged students in the College of Liberal Arts and Sciences. In this way, he has seen change happen in the inner world and has presided over change in the outside world.

William F. Cornell, M.A., TSTA, maintains an independent private practice of psychotherapy and consultation in Pittsburgh, Pennsylvania, offering frequent consultation and training programs in Europe. He has authored or edited numerous books on psychodynamic psychotherapy and somatic psychology. A coeditor of the *Transactional Analysis Journal* for 15 years, he is now the editor of the Routledge book series "Innovations in Transactional Analysis." He is the recipient of the Eric Berne Memorial Award and the European Association for Transactional Analysis Gold Medal, in recognition of his writing.

Edward T. Novak, M.A., is a psychoanalyst and maintains a private practice in Akron, Ohio. His recent book, *Physical Touch in Psychoanalytic Psychotherapy: Transforming Trauma through Embodied Practice* was published in 2023 by Routledge. He is a graduate of the National Institute for the Psychotherapies' National Training Program in Contemporary Psychoanalysis. He is the book review editor for the *Transactional Analysis Journal* and a member of the editorial board.

Michael Uebel, Ph.D., LCSW, is a researcher and mental health provider, both in private practice and with the US federal government serving military veterans. He has published on gender and sexuality issues, mindfulness, medieval thought and literature, and a wide range of psychological and psychoanalytic topics. He has been a lecturer at the School of Social Work at the University of Texas and has taught literature, women's studies, and social theory at the University of Virginia, Georgetown University, and the University of Kentucky.

Vamık D. Volkan, MD, is Professor Emeritus of Psychiatry, University of Virginia; President Emeritus of International Dialogue Initiative and past President of the Virginia Psychoanalytic Society, Turkish-American Neuropsychiatric Society, International Society of Political Psychology, and American College of Psychoanalysts.

Foreword

Sigmund Freud, in his early efforts to develop psychoanalytic theories, minimized the idea of the sexual seduction of children coming from the external world in favor of it originating from the stimuli that come from the child's own wishes and fantasies. Starting in 1925, the role of traumatic reality—actual sexual abuse—on individuals' internal worlds became the basis of a long-lasting dispute between him and the Hungarian psychoanalyst Sándor Ferenczi (Falzeder & Brabant, 2000; Paláez, 2009). In 1932, Freud's followers blocked Ferenczi from delivering a paper that focused on the truthfulness of seduction. This long dispute played a role in the path taken by other pioneer psychoanalysts, as they continued to follow Freud's path that placed less emphasis during psychoanalytic treatment on the impact of actual seduction coming from the external world and generalized this attitude to include de-emphasis on the impact of other external real events in the appearance of analysands' symptoms and character traits.

Freud and several pioneering analysts were interested in examining history, culture, religion, arts, and other shared external events from a psychoanalytic angle. But, in the clinical setting, the impact of such events on analysands' psyche was not of primary concern. Following World War I, Freud wrote about "war neurosis" and stated that he was not aware

> that patients suffering from traumatic neurosis are much occupied in their waking lives with memories of their accident. Perhaps they are more concerned with *not* thinking of it. Anyone who accepts it as something self-evident that their dreams should put them back at

night into the situation that caused them to fall ill has misunderstood the nature of dreams.

(1920, p. 13)

A few years later he described how war neuroses "opened the eyes of the medical profession to the importance of psychogenesis in neurotic disturbances, and some of our psychological conceptions, such as the 'gain from illness' and the 'flight into illness'" (Freud, 1925, p. 54). However, the emphasis on the unconscious, to a great extent, screened out the influence of external events and traumas associated with those events, especially when the patient was not an active player in an external event taking place in his or her neighborhood, community, ethnic group, or nation. The focus in the clinical setting was on exploring psychic reality only: an analysand's unconscious conflicts, resistances against exploring them, development of transference neurosis, and their resolution.

In 1932 Albert Einstein wrote a letter to Freud asking the following questions: "Is there any way of delivering mankind from the menace of war? . . . How is it possible for [a small group hungering for political power] to bend the will of the majority, who stand to lose and suffer by a state of war, to the service of their ambitions?" and "Is it possible to control man's mental evolution so as to make him proof against the psychoses of hate and destructiveness?" (Freud, 1932, pp. 199–201). In his response to Einstein, Freud expressed little hope for an end to war and violence or the role of psychoanalysis in changing human behavior beyond the individual level. In a sense, Freud provided another example that discouraged psychoanalysts from considering external events within the clinical setting, this time major tragedies linked to war and politics. There were, of course, exceptions, but they followed Freud's lead in another area that also blocked the potential influence of psychoanalysis on diplomacy and peace studies: like Freud, these writers focused on individuals' unconscious perceptions of what the image of political leaders and the mental representations of ethnic, national, religious, or ideological groups symbolically stand for (i.e.: Oedipal father, nurturing mother).

John Bowlby (1988) described that when he became an analyst in 1937, psychoanalysts in Great Britain were only interested in the internal worlds of their patients. Paying attention to historical events surrounding patients was considered inappropriate. Melanie Klein (1961) herself ignored the influences of war while treating one of her patients, a ten-year-old boy named Richard, whose analysis took place while World War II raged, literally overhead, during the London Blitz under which he and his analyst lived.

I was born in 1932 to Turkish parents on the Mediterranean island of Cyprus when it was a British colony. After graduating from a medical school in Turkey, I came to the United States in early 1957 armed with my medical degree, my violin, and only 15 dollars in my pocket, but I had a job at a hospital. I became an American citizen a few years later. My departure to the United States was part of the phenomenon known as "brain drain." The United States lacked medical doctors at this time and therefore attracted doctors from around the world. At this time the Cypriot Greeks were struggling against British rule in order to unite Cyprus with Greece. They began to oppress Cypriot Turks, as well as attacking the United Kingdom's forces and civilians. I experienced a terrible stabbing pain six months after taking up residence in America. My father sent me a newspaper clipping with very grave tidings. My roommate from the days when we lived in clapped-out lodgings in Turkey while attending the same medical school had returned to Cyprus to tend to his ailing mother. He was shot seven times and killed by a Cypriot Greek while in a pharmacy where he was buying medication for his mother. As I recall now, there was no necessary focus on the impact of such external events on my psyche while I went through my personal analysis in 1960s.

By the 1970s, American, European, Israeli, and other psychanalysts' avoidance of recalling and re-experiencing the dreadful external world of the Nazi period to a great extent had begun fading away, and more and more studies of the influence of the Third Reich on the psyche of the survivors (victims and perpetrators) surfaced. (For a review of this literature, see Brenner, 2014; Kogan, 1995; Laub & Podell, 1997; Volkan, Ast & Greer, 2002.) Anita Eckstaedt (1989) brought overdue attention to the trauma that ethnic Germans themselves experienced during the Third Reich and to the influence of that trauma on the self-conception of contemporary Germans. Judith Kestenberg's (1982) term "transgenerational transposition," Anne Ancelin Schützenberger's (1998) "ancestor syndrome," and Haydée Faimberg's (2005) description of "the telescoping of generations" referred to intergenerational transmissions of the Holocaust.

In the United States, there was an unexpected impact of psychiatrists, psychoanalysts, and other mental health professional focusing on the psychological aspects of historical events in international political, diplomatic, and military relations. On November 20, 1977, Anwar Sadat, then the president of Egypt, visited the Israeli Knesset and referred to a "psychological wall" between the Israelis and the Arabs—a wall that, he stated, accounted for 70 percent of the problems between them. Following Sadat's visit to Israel, the American Psychiatric Association's Committee on Psychiatry and Foreign Affairs, of which I was a member, brought very influential Arabs and Israelis together for unofficial dialogues once or twice a year for six years to find out if this "wall" could be made permeable. In 1988, at the University of Virginia School of Medicine, I opened the Center for the Study of Mind and Human Interaction (CSMHI). My aim was to apply a growing theoretical and field-proven base of knowledge to issues such as ethnic tension, racism, national identity, terrorism, societal trauma, leader-follower relationships, and other aspects of national and international conflict. Because no single discipline can fully illuminate such deep-seated and complex issues, CSMHI's faculty included experts in psychiatry, psychology, diplomacy, history, political science, and environmental policy. CSMHI's interdisciplinary team and I visited many areas of the world where international conflicts existed and brought together representatives of opposing large groups, such as Soviets and Americans, Russians and Estonians, Croats and Bosnians, Georgians and South Ossetians, Turks and Greeks, for unofficial dialogues. We also studied traumatized societies such as Albania and Romania after the fall of its dictators, Enver Hoxha and Nicolae Ceauşescu, respectively, and Kuwait after the invasion by Saddam Hussein's forces (Volkan, 2013). I was also a member of the International Negotiation Network (INN) under the directorship of former President Jimmy Carter for more than a decade, starting in 1989. Besides Jimmy Carter, I met other political or societal leaders such as Mikhail Gorbachev, Yasser Arafat, and Desmond Tutu and spent some time with them.

In 1980 Maurice Apprey appeared in my office with a letter of recommendation from Anna Freud. At that time, besides being the director of the Center for the Study of Mind and Human Interaction, I was the medical director of the University's Blue Ridge Hospital. Our meeting in my office was the beginning of Apprey's career at the University of Virginia. He and I had offices next to each other for many years. I got to know him closely as a friend and as a colleague and learned about his life in Ghana, Great Britain, and the United States and his exposure to different cultures and historical events. Together we taught residents of psychiatry for decades. Along with Joseph Montville, we taught diplomats at the Global Desk in the US State department how to integrate psychoanalytic thinking into their practice in 1985.

Maurice Apprey was a member of the CSMHI team when we worked in the Baltic Republics for seven years in the 1990s to help these states separate from the Soviet Union/Russia in a peaceful fashion and evolve as democratic countries. His role in our efforts was impressive, as the reader will notice from his description of some of his work in Estonia in this book. After my retirement in 2003, I was pleased to observe closely Dr. Apprey's expansion of his psychoanalytic thought into social change management at the University of Virginia in various deanship positions. I continue to admire him as a friend, teacher, and psychoanalyst and also as a strategic agent of cultural change in an organization. In this respect, one university president noted that Apprey's legacy to the University of Virginia has helped to change the culture of the entire university for the better. Another president wrote that it is rare for one person to have such a profound institutional impact.

In this book, Maurice Apprey, a psychoanalyst for children, adolescents, and adults, describes how individuals have identifications with damaged parts of internalized images of parents and illustrates how individuals, as well as ethnic, national, religious, and ideological large groups, are unwittingly possessed by historical events of their ancestors. I consider Maurice Apprey one of the most integrative thinkers for creating more knowledge about concepts of trauma, psychology of historical events, and transgenerational haunting. This important book illustrates and teaches us more about the necessity and importance of psychoanalytic study of transgenerational haunting throughout generations.

Vamık Volkan

References

Bowlby, J. (1988). *A Secure Base: Parent-Child Attachment and Healthy Human Development*. New York: Basic Books.

Brenner, I. (2014). *Dark Matters: Exploring the Realm of Psychic Devastation*. London: Karnac.

Eckstaedt, A. (1989). *Nationalsozialismus in der "zweiten Generation": Psychoanalyse von Hörigkeitsverhältnissen* [National Socialism in the Second Generation: Psychoanalysis of Master-Slave Relationships]. Frankfurt A.M.: Suhrkamp Verlag.

Faimberg, H. (2005). *The Telescoping of Generations: Listening to the Narcissistic Links Between Generations*. London: Routledge.

Falzeder, E. & Brabant, E. (2000). *The Correspondence of Sigmund Freud and Sándor Ferenczi, Vol. 3, 1920–1933*. Translated by P. Hoffer. Cambridge, MA: Harvard University Press.

Freud, S. (1920). Beyond the pleasure principle. In *Standard Edition*, Volume 18, pp. 7–64. London: Hogarth Press.

Freud, S. (1925). An autobiographical study. In *Standard Edition*, Volume 20, pp. 7–70. London: Hogarth Press.

Freud, S. (1932). Why war? In *Standard Edition*, Volume 22, pp. 197–215. London: Hogarth Press.

Kestenberg, J. S. (1982). A psychological assessment based on analysis of a survivor's child. In *Generations of the Holocaust*, eds. M. S. Bergman & M. E. Jucovy, pp. 158–177. New York: Columbia University Press.

Klein, M. (1961). *Narrative of a Child Analysis: The Conduct of the Psychoanalysis of Children as Seen in the Treatment of a Ten-Year-Old Boy*. London: Hogarth Press, 1975.

Kogan, I. (1995). *The Cry of Mute Children: A Psychoanalytic Perspective of the Second Generation of the Holocaust*. London: Free Association Books.

Laub, D. & Podell, D. (1997). Psychoanalytic listening to historical trauma: The conflict of knowing and the imperative act. *Mind and Human Interaction*, 8: 245–260.

Paláez, M. G. (2009). Trauma theory in Sándor Ferenczi's writings, 1931–1932. *International Journal of Psychoanalysis*, 90: 1217–1233.

Schützenberger, A. A. (1998). *The Ancestor Syndrome: Transgenerational Psychotherapy and the Hidden Links in the Family Tree*. New York: Routledge.

Volkan, V. D. (2013). *Enemies on the Couch: A Psychopolitical Journey through War and Peace*. Durham, NC: Pitchstone.

Volkan, V. D., Ast, G. & Greer, W. F. (2002). *The Third Reich in the Unconscious: Transgenerational Transmission and its Consequences*. New York: Brunner-Routledge.

Editor's Introduction

In Consultation, My First Meeting With Maurice Apprey

It was more than a decade ago that I first encountered Maurice Apprey's work in a book chapter, "Repairing history: Reworking transgenerational trauma," in a book of remarkable essays, *Hating in the First Person Plural*, edited by Donald Moss (2003). Apprey argued:

> In transgenerational haunting, then, a contemporary generation is unwittingly possessed by an earlier generation. The possession preserves history, but in a poisonous, un-metabolized version.
>
> (2003, p. 12)

> Accordingly, one generation of traumatized people may be so close to a trauma that they may choose never to speak about it to their children. Nevertheless, choosing to be silent does not mean that the next generation will be protected from the traumatic experience. It may, in fact, uncannily experience what it has never been told, what it seems like it never knew. The generation that is "frozen" with trauma might "inject" messages, precepts, and mandates into the next one.
>
> (p. 17)

> Self as agency is therefore an approximation; the Other as absolute is a misnomer. When Self and Other engage in the process of resolution of a conflict, a new opportunity opens up.
>
> (p. 23)

Maurice described how this silenced trauma of the previous generation is nevertheless conveyed as an urgent, unconscious "errand" for resolution. He has observed over his years of working in many different contexts of social, ethnic, and racial conflict that it is often not until the third generation

DOI: 10.4324/9781003389026-1

that these transgenerational hauntings can be brought to consciousness and addressed. Maurice's writing touched me in many ways. I found a new frame within which to begin to understand and explore traumatic aspects of my patient's histories. Inevitably, I thought of my own father returning home from World War II where he served in the North Africa and Pacific fronts. Despite his determined silence, and in fact because of his silence, the unspoken trauma of war that he brought home with him permeated— haunted—our family.

Maurice grew up in a small town in Ghana, not very far from a former slave castle that *puzzled* him as a child. The remnants and shards of unexamined histories and other historical puzzles that had hitherto remained dormant in his mind became *awakened* when, as an adult, he studied psychoanalysis under Anna Freud in London, and in the United States, studying phenomenology under Amedeo Giorgi (who incidentally had been my teacher as well in my graduate studies). In addition to his work as a psychoanalyst, Maurice has served as a full professor of psychiatry and a Dean of African American Affairs at the University of Virginia, a university that was founded in 1819 by Thomas Jefferson, a slave owner, and the original campus was built by slaves (whose names are now, finally, engraved in a memorial at the center of that first campus site). Now a man from a country that was once central to the British/American slave trade holds a high position at a university that was founded by a former slave owner in a state that had fought in the U.S Civil War to preserve slavery and had held black people as second-class citizens for another century after losing the war. Here was a man, I imagined, who knew how to make his way as a stranger in a world that must have been far less than welcoming to him. Here was a man who took one historical puzzle from one continent to another, and one academic discipline to another to navigate what "haunting" truly meant.

At the time of my initial encounters with Maurice's work, I was struggling particularly hard with one patient, Teresa, who repeatedly came to mind as I was reading. Having been deeply affected by his writing, I invited Maurice to teach a seminar on transgenerational haunting as a part of the "Keeping Our Work Alive" seminars that we sponsor in Pittsburgh for psychotherapists and psychoanalysts committed to the practice of in-depth psychotherapy. Maurice presented his model for understanding the urgent, unconscious errands imposed upon an unwitting recipient of the transgenerational "hauntings" of previous generations. He also offered a redefinition of "resistance" as an opportunity rather than only a defense.

It was a first sample of the many times he would take familiar psychoanalytic concepts and transform that into new realms of meaning. As he asks in a chapter included in this book:

> What *implications* present themselves when we use existing psychoanalytic theories in inflexible ways as points of entry into psychoanalytic exploration? What may we come to grasp if, for example, we treat some forms of resistance as opportunities rather than opposition to analytic understanding?
>
> (Apprey, 2017, p. 16)

The day-long seminar would allow time for a case consultation and the topic of the day was an ideal structure for the presentation of my work with a young woman with whom I was feeling quite useless as her therapist. I was stuck a cycle of blame—either myself as incompetent or my patient as impossibly resistant. An accounting of my that initial consultation/encounter with Maurice that day, now more than a decade ago, will serve as a vivid illustration of Maurice in action and his compassionate exploration of resistance and analytic impasse. Since that first seminar, Maurice has been a regular and deeply valued teacher in our ongoing seminars.

From the first session with Teresa, there was a sense of disturbance that seemed to reach beyond her and the problems she identified as brining her into therapy. A doctoral student in her mid-20s, Teresa was hesitant to begin therapy, having recently left a psychoanalytic therapy that had ended badly. Throughout her previous therapy, she had felt both judged and misunderstood by her female psychoanalyst. The therapy ended by mutual agreement with both Teresa and her analyst feeling defeated. As she struggled against anxiety and depression, she feared she would not be able to finish the Ph.D. program, so she decided to try therapy again, this time with a male therapist. Two years into our work together, I found myself on the edge of defeat. As much as I enjoyed and admired Teresa, there was some way in which we were both trapped in an impasse.

At our first meeting, there was, for me, an immediate contradiction in her presentation—on the one hand she was visibly, painfully shy to the degree that I felt I was supposed to look past her, while on the other hand she was dressed in a unique, highly creative style that drew my eyes with delight. It soon became clear that this contradiction was lived out in almost every aspect of her life. It appeared to me that Teresa was biracial, but there was no direct mention of it in the initial session. Her doctoral program was unusual in that it was interdisciplinary—her own creation—between English, film studies and Latino studies. She had come to Pittsburgh to pursue a Ph.D. after working several years as a documentary filmmaker, the significance of which eluded me as we began our work. The first session was dominated by stories of her distress with her previous therapist and her anxieties in her academic work, with no reference to her personal or family history.

When I inquired about her family background in the next session, Teresa said she was "bicultural," her father being Jewish and her mother Latino. She was raised as a "middle class Jew" but felt neither truly Jewish nor truly Latino. She expressed a determined disdain of both of her parents, explaining that she was actually raised by a poor, Nicaraguan woman, who was referred to in the family as grandmother, but in fact was not her grandmother. "Grandmother," who didn't speak English, raised her and was her true love object. She died when Teresa was 13, leaving this young adolescent girl bereft. Teresa felt that no one understood how profound this loss was for her. This was one of many experiences that led Teresa to develop a deeply private interior world, one that expected misunderstanding and humiliation from those around her.

From her earliest years, Teresa felt she looked neither truly Jewish nor truly Latino, "people just can't read me." This scarred her and fed her shyness as a girl, leaving her feeling like an outsider. Her older sister looked significantly more like her mother and identified as Latino. As a young girl, she was sent to intensive gymnastics lessons, accompanied by her father's fantasies of her going to the Olympics. Her father made his disappointment in her gymnastics failure well known to all. Teresa was sent to a private high school (this being right at the time that her beloved Ecuadorian "grandmother" died) that her parents could barely afford but reinforced their inflated self-images. She hated the school and what it represented but in defiance earned the highest marks. When the school day was over, she went to the Latin American cultural center that her sister attended, but she never felt she fit in the way that her sister did. Her father drove both of his daughters to be successful, to "make him proud" in his own family, who were not pleased with his choice of wife. Her childhood stories to me were dominated by accounts of her "grandmother" and her father. There was little mention of her mother, who seemed a peripheral character in the family system. By the age 16, Teresa was becoming increasingly depressed and dreamt of committing suicide. Her one reference to her mother in these initial sessions was that she told her mother of her suicidal dreams, and "there was no response." Her inner life again became more private and pained.

Teresa moved to another city to attend college. She described her college life as a "continual emotional crisis," during which she did "field research" to establish a Latino identity, immersing herself in the Latino community in her new city. She spoke only Spanish and dated a Latino guy in a relationship that she found to be good and full of emotional vitality and intensity. As we finished these initial discussions of her history and growing up experiences, she added that her current boyfriend is biracial, but "raised white." She went on to say that she didn't know how to "read the cultural signals" and no one knew how to "read" her. "I feel the scars. I feel scarred and scared."

Her family faded from our view for the next couple of years as our work was dominated by struggles in her academic work, her social anxiety, conflicted relationships with women friends, and her writing. Throughout it all, I was often taken by Teresa's piercing intelligence, which she repeatedly disowned. At some point I learned that while in college, Teresa and her Latino boyfriend produced an award-winning political documentary on life in Cuba. While Teresa might have lived this as a source of pride, instead the success was largely attributed to her partner and lived inside of her as a foreshadowing of future failure, doomed to repeatedly fall short of the mark (as in never going to the Olympics). Throughout this period, the affective intensity of Teresa's struggles dominated our sessions, but the roots and sources seemed out of our reach.

I began to feel that the therapy I had been providing up to this point had been supportive but was insufficient. I often felt more like a teacher or coach than a psychotherapist, but Teresa clearly valued our time and work together, so it had seemed "good enough." Then there was an event that shook me deeply. Teresa had written a paper that earned her a major award in her field and publication in a highly ranked journal. I hadn't even known that she had written the paper, but suddenly she was going to London to attend the major international conference in her field and receive the award. "Finally," I thought to myself, "she will be getting the recognition she deserves and won't be able to deny."

Upon her return, the first session was filled with an angry accounting of the time she spent with the woman she roomed with during the conference. I was bewildered. What about the award? Teresa reported that she said next to nothing upon receiving the award; it was as though she were paralyzed. There was a big reception afterwards, but Teresa left "vanishing without a trace," as she phrased it. Although I did not say it at the time, I thought to myself that her vanishing herself "without a trace" from an opportunity for such positive recognition must have multiple layers of meaning. I wondered what it was that was being vanished from our attention and recognition in the therapy. "Vanishing without a trace" was a phrase that took residence in my mind and became a kind of defining statement of Teresa's struggle to take her place as a competent and respected woman.

After the conference, Teresa withdrew socially and plunged into a tortured effort to write her doctoral dissertation, which became the focus of our work for the several weeks. She would spend all day in the library but end up surfing the net rather than researching or writing. When I asked her to describe in more detail what seemed to break down in her thinking and writing process, Teresa spoke at length, "I don't have a system of study. . . . I can't order my ideas. . . . Everything I write seems shitty to me. I don't know how to ask for help, total mess, humiliating to show anyone this mess. . . . I complexify everything." When I asked how she reconciled these self-perceptions with the fact that her work has already won two major awards *before* finishing her Ph.D., Teresa replied, referring to her faculty and advisors, "I wouldn't be able to survive if their opinion of me were to change in an accepting direction." I was truly taken aback by her statement, but I didn't know what to do with it. How could someone consciously court rejection and dread acceptance and recognition? She was "vanishing" her competence from the purview of her professors. I felt, too, that my own competence was vanishing.

I made the same mistake that I was beginning to realize that I was making over and over again with Teresa: I shifted our attention back to solving the problems in her writing process rather than hold on to her statement, "vanished without a trace," that had shocked me. I now recognized that I was making this mistake repeatedly in my work with her, as she seemed to be making the same mistakes over and over again in her doctoral work. But I couldn't grasp the meaning of what was happening between us. I felt locked into her tortured relationship with her mind.

In preparing for the consultation with Maurice, my anxiety was heightened by the fact that I was presenting my work in front of an important group of colleagues. I did not feel good about my work with Teresa. My frank and detailed presentation was filled with the self-criticism that had so often marked Teresa's presentation of herself and her writing. There was no criticism coming from Maurice, only a sustained, focused attention.

As I finished, he spoke to the group (reconstructed from my notes at the time):

> "I don't know Bill, as we just met this morning, but I had the very clear impression from his questions and comments during this morning's paper that he is very good at what he does. So now we have to ask ourselves the question, 'How is it that there is no evidence of that competence in the case he just presented?' That is the question for this group. How can we help Bill find the meaning of what has been happening with Teresa? There is a level of inquiry between Bill and his client that is unconsciously forbidden. Teresa, most likely without knowing that she is doing it, moves Bill repeatedly into the role of a teacher—or perhaps a father who is encouraging, demanding "success". She does not allow him to act as her psychotherapist. Her history, the history of her family is nowhere apparent. Inquiry into the past is not allowed. There are only the dilemmas of the present. It is as though this present has no past. Vanished. Banished. She has hired Bill to do a very important job, but there is a danger in this task that they have undertaken together. Here is the paradox. Bill and Teresa must examine this paradox together. Bill has asked us as his colleagues to help him burrow into this paradox. What are we to make of it?"

Maurice then invited the group to wonder aloud, to not be concerned with being right or wrong but to give voice to how the paradox was affecting them. A wise and moving discussion ensued. Maurice listened to the group, eliciting themes, and then articulated the nature of the "fundamental paradox" as he was coming to understand it.

He sat quietly for quite some time and then began to speak slowly, with long pauses between each comment, allowing space and time for me and the group to be infected and affected by his words:

> "There is an unconscious danger in shifting attention from the exterior to the interior and from the present to the past. After being given her award, Teresa disappeared herself without a trace. We have to ask ourselves, who else, what else has been disappeared without a trace. What are the traces of family tragedies, the losses that have been

disappeared? But the "traces" of these unknown tragedies remain unconscious in Teresa's struggles to define herself, to claim herself in public. What is the threat of her mixed cultural heritage? Is she to be dark or light? Is she to be middle or lower class? In her family, things aren't what they look like. Hiding, secrets, what is it that cannot be claimed? Could it be that there is something more dangerous hidden by Teresa's shyness, her disappearing of herself? She has said that she could not bear to have the faculty's opinions of her move in a positive direction. Again, I wonder, what is the danger represented by acceptance? These are the questions that must be brought into the work. Behind her incapacity to claim herself is terror, danger. We have to wonder who else has been in danger? What are the stories of the family that must be learned? She has been possessed by a phantom. She lives a problem that was not truly hers, but is now hers to face and resolve that problem together with you."

I was stunned and deeply moved. I felt as though he had opened a door that would allow me to see Teresa so differently and to begin working with her in the way she both needed and deserved. His advice to me was to "ask the questions that burrow into the paradox" and to "explore with her the family's histories for at least two generations." "She is possessed by a dilemma that is not truly hers. Your job is to help free her from the phantoms of her family, to return the phantoms to their original sources so that she can claim herself and live her own life." As I listened to Maurice, I could viscerally feel how Teresa's defensiveness and "resistance" were in fact a form of communication of the prohibitions, secrets and silences that pervaded her family.

Under the guise of doing a documentary film, they were able to talk with distant relatives of the Ecuadorian family to see if they could discover the real family history. They succeeded, learning a great deal, but at the time there was no one to help them digest it and make meaning of its consequences in their own lives. Then, ironically, when Teresa attempted to bring this history to her first therapist, she was accused of defensively shifting blame to her parents rather taking responsibility for herself. Teresa was already well accustomed to "disappearing" herself, so it had been all too easy for her to comply and disappear her history and its profound relevance yet again. For Teresa, it appeared to her that I must have agreed with her previous therapist, as I didn't inquire about her family history after the first couple of sessions. After my consultation with Maurice and my group of colleagues, I returned to my work with Teresa with a very different focus in mind. It was one that I did not expect Teresa to welcome. I was wrong. As I told her about having sought consultation and what I thought was important for us to begin wondering about together, she responded, "I think about my parents and my family constantly. I didn't think I was supposed to talk about it here." Her acquiescence to her analyst's prohibitions of speaking her family's history was deeply rooted in the family's conscious and unconscious enforced forgetting and secrets.

Suddenly, now that there was permission and space to speak them, the stories of family tragedies, lies, and secrets filled our sessions. In that seminar, Maurice argued that trauma, in and of itself, is not inherently and inevitably pathological, but that it is the lies, silence and secrets that may come to surround family trauma and tragedy that are the roots of psychopathology. As he wrote in the book chapter that first led me to invite him to our seminars:

> In transgenerational haunting, then, a contemporary generation is unwittingly possessed by an earlier generation. The possession preserves history, but in a poisonous, unmetabolized version . . . we have an obligation to learn the actual historical injury, and how it has been mentalized and extended.
>
> (2003, p. 12)

Teresa's mother's grandmother was a "black" Ecuadorian, descended from African slaves. Being "black" skinned rather than more lightly colored was enough for the family to be marginalized. Teresa told me that the "black" history of Ecuador is something that is not discussed. To intermix and intermarry with lighter skinned others was a way of moving the family into the mainstream. Teresa's grandmother had married a lighter skinned man, but he had died tragically in an automobile accident leaving his wife destitute with five daughters. Or so this had been the family story. Teresa and her sister discovered that the true story, sealed away in secrecy within the nuclear family, was that her grandmother had kicked her husband out when she learned that he had fathered a child with another woman. Grandfather then moved in with his lover whose estranged husband returned and murdered both of them in bed with a machete. Teresa's mother's family was then totally impoverished, but her mother, both very beautiful and intelligent, was awarded a scholarship to Catholic school. It was not long before the principal of the school, a priest, told her, "I will take care of you, your sisters and your family if you will become my lover." Horrified, Teresa's mother told her of the priest's offer. Teresa's grandmother told her beautiful daughter to accept the priest's generosity, so as "to let him take care of us." Teresa's mother dropped out of school, stopped being a practicing Catholic, and then moved to the United States. Emigrating to the United States allowed her to escape the horror of the life of her family, and she hoped to be able to send money home to take care of her family in a different way than the one proposed by the priest.

Once in the United States, Teresa's mother became involved in a Marxist/lesbian theater group, began writing poetry, seeking her self-respect within another marginalized community. Teresa's four aunts remained in Ecuador, all following their mother's determined message that they "marry up" into respectability and economic security. Teresa said that when she returns to Ecuador to visit her family there, her aunts are extremely controlling and absolutely "insane" about social status. Her mother was rebellious, never like her compliant, upwardly mobile sisters.

Teresa's parents met in a bar in New York. When I asked about whether there were family secrets on her father's side, she said she didn't know, but there was "lots of weird shit." Her father was "the official family fuck-up," the bad kid, constantly screwing up, constantly running out of money—a particular source of shame in a family that dearly valued money and prestige. So, Teresa's parents' marriage formed the first of many "fundamental paradoxes" that were to infect the broader family system: while her mother's marriage to a *white-skinned* American could have been a potential salvation for her family in Nicaragua, it was a disgrace and disaster to the upper middle-class intelligentsia of her father's Jewish family. For her father's family, this marriage was yet another fuck-up. Although at the same time, Teresa said to me, there was envy, "There goes Mark marrying this hot Latin chick; no Jewish woman could ever look like that." The marriage of Teresa's parents ensured that they would live at the margins of both family's cultures. Teresa said, "Both of my parents were marginalized, rebellious, troublemakers. My mother never taught my sister and I anything about manners or social behavior. She never adjusted to life in the US. She was and is treated with disdain by my father's family, so she has become a shadow of her former self."

"And then there was my father. He had violated his family's rules of race, class, and ethnicity. He wanted his kids to prove his family wrong about his mixed marriage. For us he wanted the prestige of fancy schools and fancy jobs, but neither of my parents knew how to behave appropriately in those circles. It was a mess. My father defied and mocked all social conventions. His life is a giant fuck you to the world. My mother stopped writing. As a child I loved writing, but then I would read what I wrote to my father, and he would interrupt and criticize. I stopped writing."

The parent's marriage was, and is, constantly conflicted and chaotic. Like her mother's father, Teresa's father had multiple affairs. Both daughters were and are regularly "enlisted" to side with one parent or the other during the relentless marital skirmishes. Teresa's sister was more defiant to her parents and by the time of her adolescence had created a life more distant from the family. Teresa, on the other hand, has felt a deeper sympathy, alliance and identification with her mother and has struggled with more enmeshed relationships with each of her parents. Both parents seem to Teresa to function more like perpetually defiant children than adults.

As these family stories unfolded, a very different light began to shine into my understanding of the paradoxes that permeated Teresa's life, of her careening among disparate groups and identities: Jewish, Latino, middle class, working class, Marxist, mainstream, "The Academy," community college, intelligent, stupid . . . all competing and conflicting possibilities in her mind. It became clear to me how much was a stake—the "danger" that Maurice had wondered about—for Teresa to want and to have an intelligent life for herself. The risk and dangers were held at an unconscious level, constantly distorting or destroying her own sense of choice and ownership. If she was a successful academic, was she just living out her father's dreams and demands, were these actually her father's rather than her own? If she lived a life of a successful and creative writer, was she betraying her mother, whose own intelligence and creativity that had once gained her access to a private, Catholic school and then to a theater and arts community in New York, only to be lost to a priest and then to her marriage within a Jewish family that constantly demeaned her? In our work together up to this point, we had struggled somewhat blindly within these psychological and emotional conflicts, but now we began to understand their meanings.

I wish I could write that our exploration of Teresa's family history transformed her psychotherapy. It doesn't work quite like that. What opening the doors to this history did was to help us know and feel that the depth of the conflicts Teresa felt and the urgency of them were not hers alone. Her personal struggles also bore the weight of the tragedies and unspoken violations that have permeated her family. She could not turn to her immediate family to learn a more truthful history—there was still too much investment in the secrets. Ideally, Teresa could have talked with her parents about their lives, their struggles, the broader family dynamics, and the motivations for the family secrets. But as so often the case, this was not to be.

The therapy was not magically transformed, but there were significant openings. I listened differently. I was no longer pulled to be a teacher or coach, I sat in the room as a psychotherapist. I felt the weight of the violence and violations that permeated the greater family system. I had a different sense of time. Teresa's feeling toward her parents, especially her mother, became for complex. She had often dismissed her mother as embarrassingly, hopelessly childlike. Now her mother took on the dimensions of a figure both tragic and courageous. So, too, Teresa began to inhabit a more complex and vigorous space within herself. By the time we finished therapy, she had completed a very successful doctoral thesis, married, had a child, and earned a faculty position in a prestigious university.

As is so often the case in psychoanalysis and psychotherapy, the therapeutic dyad needs to turn to a third, a consultant. Teresa and I had the very good fortune to invite Maurice into our work, and through his wisdom and interventions were then able to "invite" the conflicted and tragic voices of generations past into the room and work with us. We were able to return to the generational histories that Teresa and her sister had begun to investigate years beforehand and now imbue them with meaning and seeking to free up the present from the tragedies and demands of the past generations.

The papers gathered together here, spanning three decades of Maurice Apprey's writings, are an invitation to the psychoanalytic and psychotherapeutic communities to gain further insight and access the conflicted, tragic, and urgently pressing messages that often haunt the lives and profession of psychotherapists and the lives and hopes of our patients.

References

Apprey, M. (2003). Repairing history: Reworking transgenerational trauma. In *Hating in the First Person Plural*. Edited by Donald Moss. New York: The Other Press.

Apprey, M. (2017). Representing, theorizing and reconfiguring the concept of transgenerational haunting in order to facilitate healing. In *Transgenerational Trauma and the Other: Dialogues Across History and Difference*. Edited by Sue Grand and Jill Salberg. New York: Routledge.

Chapter 1

Delayed Preface; or, How to Read My Work

Introduction: Sources of My Earliest Intuitions; or, What I Bring From Aspects of My Development to Psychoanalysis

I am often asked mostly out of curiosity how I came to find psychoanalysis as a profession. Sometimes the enquirer wants to know how a person with multiple interests, as I have, came to choose psychoanalysis as a profession. At other times, in spite of the rich intercultural heritage in the fields of psychoanalysis, it is the curiosity of seeing a West African, in particular, in practice that gets one's attention. I hope my following remarks will feed the imagination of the reader and, at the end, see psychoanalysis in its particularity as well as grasping the interdisciplinary and intercultural praxes that it eminently possesses.

Five strands, among others, stand out as feeding sources of my coming to psychoanalysis. I touch on each of these strands as scaffolds without going deeply into anyone of them. They are meant to be simply evocative and to prepare the reader for the primary task of understanding the language deployed in this book of psychoanalytic explorations of transgenerational haunting.

First, from one side of the house in which I grew up, Fort Amsterdam, a slave castle on the coastline, the ruins of a castle built by the Dutch during the slave trade, can be seen less than a mile away. African history informs us that *bartering*, where *goods of equal value* could be *exchanged* between West Africans and Europeans, was at one time the practice between colonialists and Indigenous people. We think then of bartering in exchange of goods of equal value in West African history *as metaphor*. Enter the slave trade and its introduction of *metonymy*, where *goods of unequal value* could be transacted, as fostering an opening to the tragic view of

DOI: 10.4324/9781003389026-2

how badly humans are capable of treating each other *in a degrading and destructive way*. Paul Ricoeur (1978) follows Aristotle in this treatment of metaphors and metonymy.

If the first strand, fueled by a view from one side of my home, opened my eyes to see the difference between metaphor and metonymy, as it were, a second strand could be seen from the front of the same house where I grew up. Through the windows in front of our house can be seen a large tree some 40 to 50 yards away. It is a tree that Indigenous fetish priests would feed periodically, as if it were a god that must be fed to revitalize its soul. Like Freia's apples in Wagner's *Das Rheingold*, the gods have to eat her fruit to stay alive or else age quickly and die. Welcome to my first introduction to the tensions between the natural and the supernatural world. In these tensions, I was introduced to forms of *animism, magical thinking, cultural fetishism, totems* and *taboos* and their tensions with Christianity. Witness a telling episode in my childhood during playtime at recess when four children are chanting songs the way fetish priests and their followers would. They chant as they encircle a tree. They pretend they are going into a frenzy the way adults would. The headmaster sees them from the window of his office. He is furious. Interpreting this playful episode as a regressive transgression, he barges out of his office and chides them as follows: "Stop, boys! Don't you know that *this is exactly how you create a god*?" He is tense. The boys sheepishly return to playing harmless games like children. The headmaster, who also doubles up as the organist in our Methodist Church choir, where we sing anthems from classical music at Easter and other special occasions, returns to his office, relieved. My headmaster and Sigmund Freud would have a fascinating conversation over the classic Freudian thought that once upon a time words and magic were one and the same and that even today, words retain a decisively magical power. Accordingly, words, in Freud's psychoanalytic anthropology and metapsychology, have the power to auger well toward happiness or badly toward misfortune.

Today, I see a necessary tension between *symbolism*, where an object is itself and other than itself, and *syncretism* as a term of description in our phenomenal world where the structure of a phenomenon is embedded very, very tightly into a concrete behavior. Today, I focus largely on the multiple meanings for the subject who negotiates progressive and retrogressive steps between symbolism and syncretism.

The third strand feeds my perspective on intellectual traditions and thought as technique, following the Continental philosophers Bernard Stiegler (1998) and Ian James (2019). Here I am thinking that we can allow ourselves to have the freedom to imagine a number of epistemic conversations between different parties whose traditions of thought may otherwise be proscribed in order to reach a new sphere of influence or practice. Let us go back to my childhood to visit and to witness a lesson I learned developmentally. My father had three wives at the same time. Children having multiple parents was quite common when I was growing up. Today polygamy is illegal. In my childhood, when a father had multiple wives, their children were careful not to participate in parental disputes and tensions. The developmental task of having feuding parents whose children found ways to create meaningful and respectful relationships between them became a useful skill later in life. We heeded the implicit admonition to let parents carry on with their own fights. The implicit precept that children from multiple spouses obeyed was consequential. For us as children, then, when we play together or when we eat together, we do not have to "eat" each other. Today, this developmental freedom to not have to fight battles for parents allows me to study broadly and deeply, to think independently, and to respect the technique of thought within different traditions of psychoanalysis, phenomenology, and hermeneutics among other competing "worlds." For this reason, the so-called "controversial discussions" between Freudians and Kleinians were either techniques of thought or politics of interpretation that one could take the time to study broadly and deeply, *respectfully* paying attention to all the nuances between them, and not have to treat as dichotomies domains of thought where one tradition had to be dismissed as non-psychoanalytic. On a humorous note, let me take the reader back to my first week of training in child psychoanalysis in London. It is 1975. Every day of my first week, on my way from the Hampstead Clinic, now the Anna Freud center, to my five times weekly analysis in Chelsea, I would miss my way and end up at the Tavistock Clinic where Kleinians practiced. Call it acting out, that is, remembering in action, or motivated error, where I wished to speak to my siblings from a different parentage and in a different era, but in the United Kingdom, and in a different country, where I would surely be in danger of being blacklisted. I was saved by my analyst with one intervention after we had understood what I was doing. She said: "If you stayed with Anna Freud, you would learn many things about unconscious and conscious behaviour." She did not ever have to say more than that. For 42 years after training, I have taught psychoanalytic candidates, residents of psychiatry, medical students, psychologists, and hospital chaplains *four* traditions of psychoanalytic thought: Freud, Klein, Kohut, and Fairbairn. Today, one of my favorite intellectual activities is my participation and contributions to the *Inter-Regional Encyclopedic Dictionary* (IRED) of the International Psychoanalytic Association, the "parent" organization of multiple psychoanalytic associations with multiple languages, where the mandate of our work is not to force an integration but to represent ideas in their fullness.

The fourth strand of my coming to psychoanalysis was through the field of poetry. The poetry of W.H. Auden is the place where I got my first conceptual intuition of psychoanalytic accounts of conflict and multiple meanings, paradoxes of continuities and discontinuities within one horizon. I am referring to his poem, "On This Island," where he juxtaposes the urgent and the voluntary in a ship's errand, I address the place of this phrase in the next chapter.

Next came T.S. Eliot's *The Waste Land*, where I observed a *topographical layering* of a vertical mind and its contents. As a student of Latin and Attic Greek in middle and high school, I could not resist being glued to the epigraph that speaks of the mythic figure Sybil sitting in plain view to passersby in a vessel at Cumae, and when the boys asked her what she wanted, she answered that she wished *to die*. The question is asked in Latin; the answer is embedded in Greek. I made a mental note. This topography of mind made a distinct impression on me. I was fascinated by this craftsmanship of Petronius Arbiter—Eliot's source—of layering one idea in one language over another. Most of all, I was taken by the representation of the repression of a past mental content and the depiction of an incompatible unconscious idea within a discourse in the present unconscious.

The Four Quartets, with its exquisite accounts of *spiral circularity*, followed. I became keenly aware of comings and goings and yet remaining the same, in the same place, or creating a fresh start in order to begin a new or deferred project with a change of function. This aspect of Eliot, and not to get ahead of myself, of Freud's concepts of working through of deferred actions (nachträglichkeit) came to find a permanent place in my thinking.

The fifth strand of my coming to psychoanalysis came from classical music and Wagner in particular. In the colonial days, the Overseas Radio Service of the British Broadcasting Corporation (BBC) played classical music between the hours 8 and 10 pm before closing at 10 pm for the day. After Ghana became independent in 1957, Indigenous programming replaced the classical music program at night. This means that for the first 11 years of my life, I listened to the best of classical music at bedtime.

My good fortunes continued. I went away to boarding school at Mfantsipim Secondary School in Cape Coast, Ghana, at age 11. Mr. Fiagbezi, my first music teacher in high school, started us off with the history of classical music and key composers. He taught us about the dominant chord in particular and intervals in general. He taught when a note goes up and when it comes down, what tension a composer is trying to resolve and how, and so on. For 40 minutes, he sat in such a way that he could face us when he talked to us, and turned slightly when he played the piano to illustrate a particular movement of music. He showed us what the genius of Wagner, for instance, did with the dominant 7th. Most of all, we could share his excitement when he played the Tristan chord, and he showed us how Wagner would introduce tension between the permissible and the impermissible in *Tristan and Isolde* at the beginning of the opera and resolve that self-same tension at the very end.

He also taught us about leitmotifs as borders and, simultaneously, a necessary part of sequencing of a narrative. All of this memory was rekindled when I married a music therapist who loved the use of music dramas as conduits of material to treat mental health patients at Osawatomie State Hospital in Kansas.

Today, in my psychoanalytic praxis, Wagner's account of how *gods are inferior to us humans* has a central place in the effort *to detoxify a violent or cynical superego and its toxic errands*. If gods are inferior to us, then, we can unpack and reconfigure, *over and over again*, their constraints and prescriptions with a new agency. Hence the place of *resubjectivization* as an oneiric *exit strategy* for patients to safely leave their psychic retreats in my psychoanalytic practice.

Today, at a personal level, I use long hours of immersion in Wagnerian music for self-care. *Tristan and Isolde*, *The Ring Cycle*, and *Parsifal*, in particular, take me into lived depths of experience of loss and the symbolic return of my late wife, who was killed in a hit and run car wreck. Prematurely taken away, she can return to the illusionistic play spaces of loss and reunion, incendiary rage and consolation, redemption and rebirth, flirtation with the impermissible, and compensation in fantasy whenever I attend Wagner festivals in the United States, Russia, Germany, Australia, or Canada.

Parenthetically, I was crushed when, as an adult, I discovered that Wagner was a "bad boy," so to speak, a womanizer and a proto-fascist. However, the seeds, as it were, of the better side of him as a composer had already been planted in my cultivated garden with lots of generative perennials with different ethical imperatives.

Let us now organize my five developmental strands into some psychoanalytic precepts, texts, and contexts.

I. Pre-Texts [sic] Emerging From Cultural, Literary, and Musical Intuitions; or, How My Antecedent Lived Experiences Naturally Come to Intersect With Psychoanalytic Theories

I bring to psychoanalysis two broadly conceived and related phenomenological presences. The first is my inchoate *lived experience* in the five previous strands, and the second is my earliest *conceptual* intuitions of psychoanalysis.

Thanks to my introduction to processes of metaphor and metonymy, symbolism and syncretism, psychoanalytic concepts like transference and topographical regression, transference and temporal regression, transference and ego regression or formal regression, and regression in the service of the ego came naturally to me. The importance of constantly making progressive and retrogressive assessments could almost be taken for granted. Hence, there is no behavior that cannot *descend* from *symbolism to syncretism* and no behavior that cannot *ascend* from *syncretism to symbolism*.

Thanks to a developmental encounter with fetishistic objects, fetishistic thinking, animism, and magical thinking, there was no obstacle to psychanalytic understanding of the juxtaposition of knowing and not knowing. Thus, an infant child's struggle with the discovery of anatomical differences between the sexes and the subsequent juxtaposition of knowing and not knowing the difference was as easy to observe as it was easy to comprehend when this juxtaposition reappeared in a fetishistic pathological condition.

The cultural dimension flowed almost seamlessly into psychoanalytic thought. Between my child and adult psychoanalytic training, I taught at the University of Virginia and had the good fortune of auditing such courses of study as "From Hegel to Derrida" or "Heidegger" taught by the philosophical pragmatist Richard Rorty. In addition, and for one year, I was also a senior fellow, under Ralph Cohen, the founding editor of *New Literary History* in the English Department and the erstwhile interdisciplinary Commonwealth Center for Literary and Cultural Change. From Rorty, I welcomed his admonition to "study everything." For about five years, then, I spent my lunch hours in his graduate seminars. A philosophical pragmatism and the politics of interpretation, then, became necessary attitudes for separating and deepening complex thinking, and now it is almost second nature to say, like Rorty, "it depends . . ."

Another major influence came from my studies with Amedeo Giorgi, the renowned American phenomenological psychological researcher. He taught me the work of these thinkers from Continental philosophy: Edmund Husserl, Gaston Bachelard, and Maurice Merleau-Ponty and asked me to translate the work of Georges Politzer, the first serious critique of Freud's structural theory, written in 1928, from French into English. I followed up with the work of Heidegger, Jean-Luc Nancy, Jean Luc-Marion, and Claude Romano, among others. Out of this composite of work that is often called the reception of French thought from German philosophy came my emphasis on a Husserlian constitutive approach to psychoanalysis. Hence my interest in (1) how the subject selects particular *nodal points in one's history*; (2) how one translates *events of history* into *a sense of history* through the representational world and brings it into the room through the creation of the transference; and (3) how the subject uses the transference as a play space to *command* the analyst to repeat, witness, or reconfigure trauma or resubjectivize a set of historical grievances. Along these lines, fidelity to the mind of a subject depends on the capacity of the analyst to wait for the readiness of the subject to see the unseeable and hear the inaudible and, when necessary, to gently prod a discerning mind to go further into meaning making. Hence, description precedes interpretation; Husserl before Freud, in general.

I tested this notion that description precedes interpretation, especially in psychoanalysis, on the work of Donald Meltzer, who described his psychoanalytic work as a post-Kleinian phenomenology. In his book *Sincerity and Other Works* (1994), he made the distinction between *insincerity* and *unsincerity* [sic]. He used the term insincerity to describe the psychotic *incapacity* to present a phenomenal sense of self or object with a developmentally adaptive form of authenticity or sincerity. In Freud, Meltzer's form of *insincerity* would be proximal to *ego regression* or formal regression with *florid symptoms*. Unsincerity [sic] represented, in Meltzer's work, a tendency to *misrepresent* without the organic and regressive presentation of insincerity. He used three books written by Harold Pinter to give his account of the two phenomena of insincerity and unsincerity. He chose *The Dwarfs*, *A Birthday Party*, and *The Homecoming* for his exploration. He asked his readers to read the three books by Pinter and analyze them before reading his psychoanalytic interpretations. I did. I went further. I submitted all three texts to a Husserlian psychological research praxis, line by line, and arrived at different results from his. This difference in findings after phenomenological research is not extraordinary. Validity in this context is assessed by how any third person could see how richly the researcher went from A to B, B to C, in order to arrive at one's findings even where there is a disagreement. I knew beforehand that he was not known to graciously receive feedback that was different from his expectations. Nevertheless, Dr. Meltzer was quite upset.

I took a chance (Apprey, 1997). His response was scathing (Meltzer, 1997). I was unmoved. I asked Giorgi, who designed the praxis I used to critique his work, to guide me in responding to Meltzer. This time I received no written response. We met for the first time in person at a conference on his work in Florence, Italy, two years later. In a Q and A session, I repeated my criticism of his work as much too hurried and precipitous to be correctly described as a phenomenology or even as a post-Kleinian phenomenology, as he liked to describe his psychoanalytic explorations. I offered my justifications for arriving at my conclusions. The room was quiet. I received a gentle tap on the shoulder. I turned around. It was Dr. Meltzer. He said: "You must be Dr. Apprey." During the break he shook my hand vigorously and said: "Young man, carry on!" We parted company. He died shortly after our meeting, and so we did not have the opportunity to follow up in a more meaningful way the dialogue on Husserlian phenomenology and post-Kleinian phenomenology I had hoped for. What a loss!

Earlier in my career, Eleanor Galenson, a first-rate developmental psychoanalyst, had used the same words Dr. Meltzer used to congratulate me after a panel presentation on incest at a Margaret Mahler Symposium in Philadelphia, Pennsylvania: "Young man, carry on!" Fortified by the blessing of these two analysts that I respected immensely, I soldiered on, maintaining orthodoxy and recreating in a plastic way my philosophically pragmatic and nuanced renditions. In the spirit of Gaston Bachelard, the way to debunk an idea is to start with it and then systematically depart from it. I am not quite so radical. So, sometimes, I follow another stream of his thought that suggests that synthesis is transformation. Still following Bachelard, instead of dichotomies, I want to *create complementarities out of antinomies*. Like Richard Rorty, the quintessential philosophical pragmatist, what praxis I use *depends on* my current project.

In another vein, especially in my account of a psychoanalytic process, and following Deleuze (1988), inside and outside *fold* into each other. Instead of circularity, then, I consider *spiral circularity*.

In the course of my international education, then, I have welcomed the opportunities to study broadly and deeply. However, as a psychoanalyst, I do have an anchor: Freud's metapsychological papers from 1914–1923 and Freud's papers that speak to his work as a cultural theorist.

II. Representative Texts for Interrogating Conceptual Pretexts in Psychoanalysis

The texts I use to anchor my work, especially when I teach, are Freud's metapsychological papers. For some 16 years I was a member of an international faculty that created a psychoanalytic institute in Istanbul, an institute that recently received its full accreditation and became a component member of the International Psychoanalytic Association. For 16 years I taught nothing but these metapsychological papers: *The Unconscious* (1914), *Instincts and Their Vicissitudes* (1915a), *Repression* (1915b), *Beyond the Pleasure Principle* (1920), and *The Ego and the Id* (1923).

I taught these texts for five hours on Saturdays and clinical seminars for five hours on Fridays and Sundays, four full weekends a year. The immersion was total.

For my projects on psychoanalytic anthropology, in other contexts, these three texts by Freud were most useful to me: *The Future of an Illusion* (1927), *Totem and Taboo* (1913), and *Civilization and Its Discontents* (1930). I read *The Future of an Illusion*, for instance, along with Winnicott's "Transitional Objects and Transitional Phenomena" (1951), Paul Pruyser's *A Dynamic Psychology of Religion* (1968), *Between Belief and Unbelief* (1974), *The Play of the Imagination* (1983), and *The Minister as Diagnostician* (1976), in order to teach clinical pastoral education to hospital chaplains in training at the University of Virginia.

The University of Virginia was a fountain of interdisciplinary studies when I joined the faculty in 1980, and it is still somewhat the case in spite of current economic pressures, relative self-serving interests and obligations within departments, and changing times. In any case, it was very common to be invited to guest teach a course in other departments or serve as a reader on dissertation committees in departments of English, anthropology, religious studies, and others. Victor Turner, the cultural anthropologist who wrote about liminality and limonoid spaces, had recently passed away before I came to Virginia. However, his wife, Edie Turner, invited me to co-teach a graduate anthropology seminar with her on healing by means of imaginary forms of "tooth extraction" in a village she had studied during her anthropological field work. Here, we studied what Pruyser called the "illusionistic world" as play space. Accordingly, between the autistic world and the realistic world, there lies the world of tutored fantasy in that intermediary third world. Between untutored fantasy and sense perception, there lies the world of tutored fantasy. Between the domain of symptoms and signs, there lie symbols. Between hallucinatory entities and actual entities, there lie imaginative entities or events.

My paper "Liminality as Metaphor in Adolescent Psychotherapy and Psychoanalysis" (Apprey, 1987) was written during that period.

III. From Pretexts and Texts to Context of This Book

Finally, and focusing on this book alone, on toxic errands through the generations, I am undertaking a conceptual transformation of Freud's concept of the four properties of an instinct. In Freud, an instinct has a source. It operates under pressure. It has an active and a passive aim. It has an object through which desire is to be attained.

Following Bachelard, every biological template has a psychological correlate. Every materiality has a functional correlate.

When we go from two generations to three generations to define a subject, we get the following. The source of an instinct exceeds biology. Ancestral influences prevail. Embodied imperatives are passed on through identification and other means. Instinctual trends therefore have a long history, and they enter the representational world of the subject in a slow and insidious way. In such a world, active and passive alternate, and they do so in ways where subject as object of an other's desire to carry out a mandate shall have lost sight of the origin of the toxic errand. A middle voice happening devoid of active and passive shall have taken over.

One's sense of time shall have changed. A pluperfect tense replaces that which resembles a linear or even a circular sense of time. By the time subject shall have recognized that one is a captive, the toxic errand shall have already taken place.

Something has been deferred in a process Freud called nachträglichkeit. Subject now lives in a suspended haunt of a representational world. In treatment, clinician and patient must now co-create a generative setting where history can be reconfigured in the present unconscious so that an exit strategy to advance one's psychological freedom can be designed and fostered.

So, at the end of the day, what is in an *errand*? A *mandate* to carry out a pro-ject [sic] that is not originally one's own? Is an errand *a wondering away* from one's own journey? Who *errs* when a subject is sent away? How does a subject who goes on an errand *return*? Changed? Unchanged? Whose poison does a subject carry *across* generations? Who *urgently* infuses a toxic errand? How does one *voluntarily*, preconsciously or unconsciously, pick one's own poison, as one transports the poison from an anterior place into one's own *version*, in one's *turn*? What kind of work does a clinician do with an analysand, *a fellow seeker*, as it were, to *reconfigure* the appropriated transgression? What psychoanalytic attitude does one adopt to facilitate the psychoanalytic process? How faithful can an analyst be to a patient's *constitutive* mind in the psychoanalytic process? How does the subject create *an exit strategy* of one's own to secure one's freedom from psychological captivity?

These are some of the questions in my psychoanalytic explorations of the phenomenon of transgenerational haunting. I hope that these explorations will feed the imagination of other clinicians as they embark on making meaning in ways that exceed the *limits* posed by psychopathology, dysfunctional behavior, trauma, or whatever brings a patient to see a clinician.

Besides patients who are fellow seekers in my work, there are others who think with me. Clinicians who seek consultations are eminent partners in learning more about transgenerational transmission and other phenomena. This book strategically positions two such consultations, written by two seasoned clinicians, as borders.

Finally, because there are other explorations that border on the current subject of transgenerational haunting and other encounters in my work, I have added other papers that indicate how I variously situate myself in the world as a clinician; a phenomenological psychological researcher; and teacher of medical students, residents of psychiatry, psychoanalytic candidates, and others.

References

Apprey, M. (1987). Liminality as metaphor in adolescent psychotherapy and psychoanalysis. In *From Metaphor to Meaning: Papers in Psychoanalytic Anthropology*, eds. H. F. Stein & M. Apprey, pp. 94–109. Charlottesville & London: University of Virginia Press.

Apprey, M. (1997). When disciplined description precedes interpretation: Slowing down Meltzer's account of *Sincerity* to reinsert description in post-Kleinian phenomenology. *Journal of Melanie Klein and Klein Object Relations*, 15(1): 91–130.

Deleuze, G. (1988). *The Fold: Leibniz and the Baroque*. New York: Continuum Press.

Freud, S. (1913). Totem and taboo. In *Standard Edition*, Volume 13, pp. 1–162. London: Hogarth Press, 1953.

Freud, S. (1914). The unconscious. In *Standard Edition*, Volume 14, pp. 159–215. London: Hogarth Press, 1957.

Freud, S. (1915a). Instincts and their vicissitudes. In *Standard Edition*, Volume 14, pp. 109–140. London: Hogarth Press, 1957.

Freud, S. (1915b). Repression. In *Standard Edition*, Volume 14, pp. 141–158. London: Hogarth Press, 1957.

Freud, S. (1920). Beyond the pleasure principle. In *Standard Edition*, Volume 18, pp. 1–64. London: Hogarth Press, 1957.

Freud, S. (1923). The ego and the id. In *Standard Edition*, Volume 19, pp. 3–66. London: Hogarth Press, 1961.

Freud, S. (1927). The future of an illusion. In *Standard Edition*, Volume 21, pp. 3–56. London: Hogarth Press, 1961.

Freud, S. (1930). Civilization and its Discontents. In *Standard Edition*, Volume 21, pp. 59–145. London: Hogarth Press, 1961.

James, I. (2019). *The Technique of Thought*. Minneapolis, MN: University of Minnesota Press.

Meltzer, D. (1994). *Sincerity and Other Works*. London: Karnac Books.

Meltzer, D. (1997). Reply to Maurice Apprey's paper. *Journal of Melanie Klein and Object Relations*, 15(1): 131–132.

Pinter, H. (1959). *The Birthday Party*. New York: Grove Weidenfeld.

Pinter, H. (1961). The dwarfs. In *Harold Pinter: Complete Works*, Volume 2. New York: Grove Weidenfeld.

Pinter, H. (1965). The homecoming. In *Harold Pinter: Complete Works*, Volume 3. New York: Grove Weidenfeld.

Pruyser, P. (1968). *A Dynamic Psychology of Religion*. New York: Harper and Row.

Pruyser, P. (1974). *Between Belief and Unbelief*. New York: Harper and Row.

Pruyser, P. (1976). *The Minister as Diagnostician: Personal Problems in a Pastoral Perspective*. Philadelphia, PA: The Westminster Press.

Pruyser, P. (1983). *The Play of the Imagination: Toward a Psychoanalysis of Culture*. New York: IUP.

Ricoeur, P. (1978). *The Rule of Metaphor: Multidisciplinary Studies of the Creation of Meaning in Language*. London & Henley: Routledge and Kegan Paul.

Stiegler, B. (1998). *Technics and Time 1: The Fault of Epimetheus*. Palo Alto, CA: Stanford University Press.

Winnicott, D. W. (1951). Transitional objects and transitional phenomena: A study of the first not-me possession. *International Journal of Psychoanalysis*, 34: 89–97.

Chapter 2

The Urgent and the Voluntary in Errands

W.H. Auden and My Very First Intuitive Grasp of Psychoanalysis

When I was a student at The Anna Freud Centre, I marveled at the way Anna Freud responded to a paper that a student or a member of the teaching faculty had taken months to write. In a ten-minute discussion, she would give a crisp account of the metapsychology behind the intrapsychic story of the case in a most engaging way. I wanted to learn how to do that. In her story making technique, *description invariably preceded interpretation*. It was an intuition then. Now, and for the first time, I know that one can train oneself to emulate that.

Another aspect of her functioning was her philosophical pragmatism. While others debated the merits of the topographical theory or the structural theory and/or their continuities and discontinuities, she would say the following:

> Different from the people who found the structural theory in existence when they entered psychoanalysis and saw the topographical scheme as a thing of the past, I grew up with the topographical scheme, and had a gradual transition to the structural in my own psychoanalytic development. I must say that. . . . I never made the sharp distinction between the two that later writers made, but according to my own convenience I used the one or the other frame of reference.
>
> (Sandler with Anna Freud, 1985)

Now, and for the first time, I have come to grasp the continuities between the two systems as indices of *structural delay.* First, selections from the sedimentations of history get appropriated by the subject. Second, the appropriations come to create a representational world. Third, out of this representational world, transference wishes, pleas, and demands enter the public space of the analytic setting between the patient and the analyst.

DOI: 10.4324/9781003389026-3

The intentionality behind the wishes, pleas, or demands requires reciprocal connection and reciprocal correction to enable hitherto unresolved grievances, conflicts, or deficits to be negotiated and renegotiated until a reconfiguration of the subject's world shall have taken place. The most representative account of my work using this frame of reference is in a special issue on intercultural analysis in the January 2006 issue of *The Psychoanalytic Quarterly*. It is reprinted in this book as Chapter 6.

How does this structural delay between the topographical and the structural schema show itself? What is the nature of the relationship between internal fields of reference to the outside and, in reverse, external fields of reference to the inside? How is it that a parent has parents, and yet we focus inordinately on the primary caregiver and the child? Where do generations fit into the work of psychoanalysis? These and other transformations into what we know as the psyche have preoccupied me for years.

Some of these questions have been answered. In Andre Green (2000), we learn that in a structural delay, the "paradise" of the mother-infant relationship translates into the "id." The relationship of a mother to her mother translates into the "ego." The "superego" is the end product of the father's role that ends the two-in-one relationship between the mother and her baby to which she is bodily linked. In the translation of the father's role into the formation of the superego, Green indicated that time brings a sense of order and registers prohibition in order to declare that the child is in a different generation from the father. *Two generations are therefore not sufficient to define a human subject, and it takes at least three to do so because even in the mother-child relationship, there is the potential idea of the father inside the mother and the father outside the mother.* In other words, in Green's praxis, the timelessness of the unconscious brings up the imperative of the paternal function to provide order, generalization, and continuity.

The idea of three generations in psychoanalysis is not new. Providing an adaptational view, Heinz Hartmann (1958, p. 30) wrote that the human subject does not come to terms with its environment anew in every generation. Rather, this relation to the environment is guaranteed by an evolution peculiar to us humans through the influence of tradition and the survival of our creations. Accordingly, we take over from others a great many of our methods for solving problems. We therefore live in past generations as well as in ours.

Since Hartmann we have gone much further in describing multi-generational transactions. Haydee Faimberg (2005), Vamık Volkan (2002), and Apprey (1993b) have described different ways in which the ego can be subject to tyrannical intrusions, and it happens in ways that cause the subject to carry mandates of intrusive parental projects with which the ego may identify and appropriate as one's own. *My theoretical interest in this unconscious transfer between subject and object dates back to age 15.* It was a time when I had not yet learned that a student must have empathy for teachers who were trying to do their best. In a literature class, my Latin teacher, who also taught the poetry of W.H. Auden, described the juxtaposition of the urgent and the voluntary in errands in the poem "On This Island" as an *oxymoron*. I protested that his rather cavalier attempt at interpreting the phrase from Auden lost sight of a powerful *metaphor* that depicts human conflict. I intuited then that the urgent and the voluntary can coexist in one metaphor. Today, I see an *urgently infused mandate* being given, a mandate *followed by a voluntary appropriation*. This appropriation gets mentalized and undergoes a structural delay. Subject and object shall have changed places so that the subject now has his or her own poison to deliver, as it were. Now, and for the first time, I realize how formative that argument with my Latin teacher who had doubled as a teacher of English literature was. Now I write about maternal *misconception, transgenerational haunting, dreams of urgent voluntary errands,* among other notions of psychical transfer and appropriations into the domain of the representational world.

Two opportunities allowed me to advance my work on psychical transfer from here: one from psychoanalysis, the other from Continental philosophy. From psychoanalysis, I encountered Robert Stoller's work. From my study of French reception of Husserl's philosophy, I studied closely Descartes, Foucault, Bachelard, Merleau-Ponty, Politzer, and Romano, among others.

From psychoanalysis, I was particularly intrigued by Stoller's account of a mother whose nine-year-old son wanted to become a girl. (Stoller, 1968). The mother spoke about her relationship with her mother before she bore a son. She felt like a cipher. She hoped to become a nun. Notice what the word "nun" sounds like. Her recurrent dream before she had a son was as follows: "I had died and was now dead. But my mother kept sending me to the store on errands because she had not even paid enough attention to know it". This case and Stoller's interpretation of a mother's emptiness and a grandmother's refusal to lend her femininity to her daughter, resulting in massive object hunger in a mother, along with a persisting bisexuality, did not constitute an epiphany for me. Rather, I felt I had confirmation for an idea that needed to be further developed.

From Continental philosophy, I came to assemble the following ideas about the human subject as follows. From Descartes we could say, with some qualification, that the human subject is realized through its encounter with "*truth*" and with indubitable certainty. The human subject in Foucault is realized through its encounter with "*errors*": errors as *mistakes, wanderings,* preconscious or unconscious representations of *mandates.* In Husserl the researcher constitutes intersubjective phenomena *without presupposition* and in the service of *fidelity to the perceived object.* We travel then *from the events of history to a sense of history* as we create intersubjective constitution of perceived phenomena. In Claude Romano, the subject that constitutes phenomena in Husserl is now radicalized so that *the subject is one who comes back to oneself, an* "*advenant*" (Romano, 2009).

Various syntheses of ideas from both psychoanalysis and Continental philosophy enabled me to rethink Freud's account of the four properties of instincts. At one time, I thought of an instinct as having a biological *source,* as operating under *pressure,* as having an *aim,* and as having an *object.* Now I think as follows: beyond biology, an ancestral mandate with a peremptory wish is formulated; the unconscious wishes behind that mandate undergo structural delay so that they lose their urgency and are instead suspended; active injection and obedient reception change places; agency between subject and object alternate. Finally, the object through which the satisfaction is to be derived is but a figuration in the representational world; an introjected self, as it were.

The result of this reframing of Freud has made me so glaringly aware that we often think we are experientially going somewhere only to realize that we have *already* been there. Or we think we have a project only to realize that we have already been *sent.*

Thus psychoanalytic time construed as timeless may no longer be demarcated as past, present, and future but rather as *pluperfect time* (Apprey, 2014).

My synthesis of ideas that subserve psychical transfer, transgenerational transmission of destructive aggression, follows that of Gaston Bachelard to this effect: synthesis is transformation. My synthesis of Auden, Freud,

Husserl, Foucault, and Romano, among others, has enabled me to coin the term "pluperfect" errand.

The idea of pluperfect errand here elaborates and brings fullness to Freud's notion of "nachträglichkeit" that translates as "deferred action." We now have a circular, ten-fold mnemic taxonomy of the nachträglichkeit behind transgenerational transfer of destructive aggression. First, a destructive ancestral mandate is formulated when a traumatized family, community, or group is attempting to change events of history into a sense of history. They must find a hospitable home for the psychological toxin. They must inject it into a suitable object. Second, and through structural delay, the injected poisonous project undergoes storage for an indeterminate period of time. Third, the indeterminate time for the storage is numinously suspended. Fourth, it is suspended until an errand can stealthily rob the carrier of one's sense of agency. Fifth, a paradox occurs where we have an urgent voluntary errand. Sixth, the subject that carries her inheritance as though it were one's own must find a new context to create a public space for reactivation, away, from the haunt, as it were. Seventh, any sense of having been sent is by now totally lost. Eighth, the categories of active and passive are now fixed in irreversible and *unrepresentable* presentations. Ninth, precisely because the infusion is unrepresentable, active or passive voices are inaudible. Finally, a middle voice must now be nurtured and co-created through *reciprocal connection* and *reciprocal correction* through the therapeutic story.

When I have presided over an analysis in this way, the unconscious errand shows itself. Now, and for the first time, I can see that ordinary and extraordinary phenomena reveal themselves through a relatively simple word like "errand," even if it is subserved by metapsychological and philosophical assumptions that have to be bracketed and suspended so that I do not get ahead of the patient.

References

Apprey, M. (1993a). Projective identification and maternal misconception. In *Intersubjectivity, Projective Identification and Otherness*, eds. M. Apprey & H. Stein, pp. 76–101. Pittsburgh: Duquesne University Press.

Apprey, M. (1993b). Dreams of urgent/voluntary errands and transgenerational haunting in transsexualism. In *Intersubjectivity, Projective Identification and Otherness*, eds. M. Apprey & H. Stein, pp. 102–130. Pittsburgh: Duquesne University Press.

Apprey, M. (2014). A pluperfect errand: A turbulent return to beginnings in the transgenerational transmission of destructive aggression. *Free Associations: Psychoanalysis and Culture, Media, Groups, Politics*, 66: 15–28.

Faimberg, H. (2005). *The Telescoping of Generations*. New York: Routledge.

Green, A. (2000). *Andre Green at the Squiggle Foundation*. London: Karnac Books.

Hartmann, H. (1958). *The Ego and the Problem of Adaptation*. New York: IUP.

Romano, C. (2009). *Event and World*. New York: Fordham University Press.

Sandler, J. with Freud, A. (1985). *The Analysis of Defense: The Ego and the Mechanisms of Defense Revisited*. New York: IUP.

Stoller, R. (1968). *Sex and Gender*. New York: Jason Aronson.

Volkan, V. (2002). *Third Reich in the Unconscious*. New York: Routledge.

Chapter 3

Repairing History
Reworking Transgenerational Trauma

The idea of intercultural psychoanalysis, community psychiatry, or any expression of cross-cultural mental health has many pitfalls that have to be worked through. The effort to understand cross-culturally and to repair the ravages of historical injuries requires at the very least a disclosure of one's basic assumptions, an ethic of translation, and a series of well-considered praxes for intervention. This is particularly so when hatred and violence are implicated in the object of study and/or intervention. If this triad of basic assumptions, translation, and praxes is well modulated, new descriptions of self and other are likely to emerge. This chapter, then, will serve as a catalogue of issues that subserve an approach to the work we do in the field of transforming the impact of history in transgenerational trauma so that change may become possible.

Operational Format of This Chapter

The operational format of this chapter begins with an ethic of translation that is involved in any account of cultural transmission. What is *carried over* when we tell a story? What is *betrayed* along the way? Second, as we cross over from one generation to the next, what do we take over from the previous generation and what vicissitudes of change take place? Third, when we cross over to the next generation, what fades away as a sedimentation of history and what is selectively reactivated and subsequently extended to serve new and contemporary purposes? Fourth, how do we store cultural memory and what is the consequence of the *mode of storage* on the actual form of transmission of cultural memory? Fifth, the form of storage and reactivation ranges from a concrete, syncretic form to the symbolic. Sixth, *syncretic, amovable*, and *symbolic* forms have consequences for practice. Seventh, as we differentiate the syncretic, amovable,

DOI: 10.4324/9781003389026-4

and symbolic forms of expression, we can differentiate toxic errands. Last, we can transition from individual work to group work. The chapter on "containing the uncontainable" gives us a slice of how group work may be done in intercultural or ethno-national psychoanalysis.

I. Inserting an Ethical Dimension Into the Repair of Transhistorical Trauma: Translation as Carry-Over and/or Betrayal

Before I go further, allow me to feed your imagination with three anecdotes on translation as a carry-over and/or as betrayal depending on the context.

At a recent annual conference of the Association of Child Psycho-Analysis, I found myself accosted by three colleagues, one of them African American, the other two Jewish Americans. Each was sympathetic to the protest of some African American clinicians who had heard the term *chosen trauma* used by my colleague, Vamık Volkan. The conversation went as follows:

"You work with Vamık Volkan, don't you?"
"Yes I do."
"What does he mean by 'chosen' trauma?"
"It's about how the events of history are changed into a sense of history by a victimized group and mentalized in ways that subsequently come to define their cause."
"That's not good enough. It's narrow and incomplete, and for African Americans, in particular, it's like doing violence to them by neglecting the violence done to them in their history."

The conversation was not long enough for me to elaborate on or address the current of human feelings aroused in them by the term *chosen trauma*. Subsequently we have maintained a continuing successful dialogue about the process of conceptualizing the experiences of traumatized groups. These three colleagues can now agree that no concept is sufficient in capturing the experiences of all traumatized groups, and therefore discretion is required in the process of translation.

The second anecdote comes from an encounter with a Jewish American candidate, a recent immigrant from Israel, in a seminar that I led on cross-cultural issues in psychoanalysis. Usually, when I lead this seminar at this particular institute, I ask members to give a brief account of their ethnic origins, and we discuss the role their origins plays in their practice of psychoanalysis. Typically, they learn more about each other than they had ever imagined. On this one occasion, I made the error of going straight to the cognitive content of the course and paid dearly for it. Quite soon after the seminar began, I found myself illustrating the difference between metaphor and metonymy by providing examples from mass grave sites for Jews in Lithuania, Latvia, and Estonia, As I spoke, I saw one candidate fuming. Why had I chosen those examples? Who did I think I was to talk about those sites? In her view, I was much too polished to have suffered in life. To be precise, I hadn't suffered enough to have earned the right to speak about such issues. After some deliberation I recovered my poise and returned to my usual format of beginning the seminar with process material and allowing the discussion of theory to emerge out of the discourse. I was not invited back again.

In the third anecdote, an African American woman said to me, after hearing a paper on transgenerational trauma, "Thank you for not pathologizing us. I hope in the course of your work you'll do another paper on the perpetrators of hatred and violence on African Americans to give us a balance." She was right. I came to appreciate that an ethic of translation that includes human motivation from the side of transgressors as well as from the side of the transgressed in cross-cultural discourse on community psychoanalysis must not be overlooked.

In the first anecdote, I was *guilty by association*. In the second, *I did not prepare the candidates at the emotional level* before I proceeded to the course content. In the third, *I was affirmed for not wounding my audience*, precisely because what one intends is not necessarily how one's message is received. An ethic of translation, then, is called for.

What would an ethic of *translation* be? It is the recognition that ideas can *carry over* from one place to another, sometimes well, sometimes badly. It is the recognition that the formulation of theory can also be received as *betrayal* of those very transgressed people we wish to describe. These two meanings of translation as a *carry-over* and translation as *betrayal* require us to be circumspect as clinicians, researchers, and theorists. Care is needed to understand that when one describes or interprets, there is invariably *opposition* involved. There is opposition of one's desire to translate against the desire of another person about whom the translation is being conducted.

We would do well then to consider our theoretical formulations as pro-visional, idiomatic, and never wholly satisfactory, thus ensuring that our theoretical formulations do not injure the other. One way of ensuring that we do not needlessly injure the very group whose experience of trauma we intend to address is by allowing description that is faithful to the mind of the transgressed to precede interpretation. In a *particular* description of a traumatized ethnic group, we may do well to treat that which looks like an exception as a *profile* of human behavior. In this way we get to freeze that which looks like an exception long enough to see ourselves in it. Thus, a Native American subject, for instance, who finds a psychological test much too intrusive requires an *open-ended* interview to begin to elicit pertinent clinical information. This example tells us less about Native Americans, in se, than it tells us that all clinicians must learn to be skilled open-ended interviewers for *all subjects*, always sensitive to issues of intrusion. Who among us humans, outside the particularity of an Indigenous group, cannot benefit from well-crafted open-ended interviews?

The notion, then, that the exceptional is but a profile reduces the awk-wardness of translation of ideas that so often plagues cross-cultural writ-ings. In this respect, the adverse consequences for African Americans that are the result of slavery and Jim Crow laws are not necessarily particular to African Americans. However, they will highlight some general human phenomena that I want to emphasize in the realm of difference and iden-tity. In short, we can start with the particular and depart from it.

II. Introducing Transgenerational Haunting and the Pivot of Difference and Identity

Manifestations of violent ethnonational conflicts are inseparable from his-tory. Invariably, these forms of conflict are subserved by the shift *from how humans translate the events of history to a contemporary sense of history*. In this respect we are dealing with *appropriations of history*. The psychoanalyst Heinz Hartmann (1958) spoke to this issue of appropriation in ways that are consistent with my understanding of historical transfor-mations: people do not come to terms with the environment anew in every generation; their relation to the environment is guaranteed by an evolution peculiar to humans: the influence of tradition and the survival of the works of humankind. *We take over from others a great many of our methods for solving problems*. The works of humans objectify the methods they have discovered from solving problems and thereby become factors of continu-ity, so that *humankind lives*, so to speak, *in past generations as well as in their own* (p. 30).

In addition to the transgenerational transmission of destructive agg-ression, I want to suggest that the appropriations of history have some very specific contents. With respect to violent ethnonational conflicts, the pivotal issues are *difference* and *identity*. It is as if humans had an obligation, albeit self-imposed, to cleanse ourselves of some inchoate and un-metabolized parts of ourselves which we dare not admit belong to us and must therefore be housed elsewhere, or worse, deposited to the world of *no place*, namely *death of the Other*. Introducing transgenera-tional haunting and difference/identity, I want to think of the transgen-erational as the vertical axis and issues of difference and identity as occupying the place of the horizontal axis. Within the realm of the verti-cal there lie the events of history that undergo a change of function from one generation to the other. Within the realm of the horizontal there lies the modern-day drama of configuring the events of history into lived contemporary drama.

Before spelling out precisely how humans live in the past as well as in the present and what they do with the Other to purify themselves and to render the Other inferior, useless, or dead, I want to plot a trajectory of how the events of history become appropriated as a sense of history. I shall, following the German literary theorist Wolfgang Iser (1992), speak of this process as *staging*.

III. Staging and Transforming Historical Grievances: The Sedimentation and Reactivation of Cultural Memory

The Estonian semiotician Yurij Lotman and his co-worker, B.A. Uspensky (1971), defined culture as "the nonhereditary memory of a community, a memory expressing itself in a system of constraints and prescriptions" (p. 411). They connected culture to past historical experience by treating culture as a social phenomenon and specifically as a memory and record of what a community has experienced. Culture then "is only perceived ex post facto" (p. 411). To be precise, "When people speak of the creation of a new culture, they are inevitably looking ahead; that is, they have in mind that which they presume will become a memory from the point of view of the reconstructable future" (p. 412). In his *Cartesian Meditations*, the German philosopher Edmund Husserl (1929) wrote of the dialectic between sedimentation (fading) and reactivation (recall) and the strategy of *reducing historical fact to a sense of and a reconstitution of that historical fact*. Ernesto Laclau (1990), an Argentinean political scientist, echoing Husserl, wrote of the shift from historical givens to *new conditions of possibility*. Along similar lines, Iser (1992) built on the work of the later Husserl to articulate his notion of staging as lived anthropological category rather than as a reflected epistemological category. Staging, for Iser, "must always be preceded by something to which it has to give appearance" (p. 885). He continues:

> This "something" can never be completely covered by the staging, because otherwise staging itself would become its own enactment. In other words, every staging lives on what it is not. For everything that materialized in it stands in the service of something absent, which, although given presence through something else that is present, cannot be present itself. Staging is thus an absolute form of doubling, not least because it always retains awareness that this doubling is ineradicable.
>
> (p. 885)

According to Iser, staging makes a separation between a *historical* given and its *new* presentation. Staging separates the historical mode from the new something that is to be given appearance. Staging then encompasses past and present. It links a historical absence to a concrete contemporary presence. It binds a conceptual given to that given's simulacrum.

Iser's concept of staging traces the journey from cultural memory through recall and from recall through the transformation of historical grievances into praxis. With the language of the French phenomenologist Maurice Merleau-Ponty (1983) in *The Structure of Behaviour*, I shall nuance this transformation and how embedded it becomes into three phenomenological prototypes when I describe storage and transformations of structures of experience in the following as syncretic, amovable, and symbolic. These three phenomenological categories of syncretic, amovable, and symbolic will give us a handle on the limits and possibilities of overturning embedded historical grievances.

IV. Some Specific Modes of Storage and Transformation of Cultural Memory: Anticipating Praxis

In order to overturn destructive appropriations of history, a heuristic approach for unmasking originary but persistent historical mandates must be undertaken. By heuristic, I mean a set of pre-theoretical ideas that can be tested in the field, given up if they do not work, and stabilized into theory if they can be shown to merit serious consideration. By *originary* and *persistent mandates*, I am referring to the mandate to preserve, let us say, an originary legacy of ashes in new but equally destructive forms. *It is as if the motor of destruction remains the same but the license plate changes.*

I am implicitly referring here to the psychoanalytic notion of change of function. Of *change of function*, Hartmann (1958) writes: "What defensive operations were anchored in instincts may subsequently be performed in the service of and by means of the ego, though naturally, new regulations too will arise in the course of development of the ego and the id" (p. 49). He continues: "Differentiation progresses not only by creation of new apparatuses to master new demands and new tasks, but also and mainly by new apparatuses taking over, on a higher level, functions which were performed by more primitive means" (p. 50). Change of function can manifest itself in destructive ways, such as murder in one generation, suicide in the next. Or it can manifest itself in a higher form when the next generation has worked through and modified destructive aggression into a sublimated means of survival.

Let us now look at four specific means of rupture and storage of cultural memory. Appropriating Hillis Miller (1992), I have suggested a four-step heuristic strategy (see Apprey, 1999) to observe and ultimately transform received hatred from an Other group. These four rubrics are related, but they are separated here in order to effect greater clarity. The key rubrics of the heuristic strategy are: (1) *line*; (2) *character*; (3) *anastomosis*, which I translate hereafter into my praxis as *transgenerational haunting*; and (4) *figure*.

Under the rubric of *line*, we may think of a broken line, a cut, an incision, a gap, or a rupture. Representative of this notion of line might be the sense of lost ancestry manifested as an absence in African American lineage. *Into this cut, as it were, may be inserted a world of lived experience where the oppressed has lost sight of the original enemy.* Influenced by this absence, a people may attack its own, as in Black-on-Black crime.

Under the rubric of *character* (from the Greek word *Kharassein*, to brand) we may think of a *scratch into the skin*, the verbs to *engrave*, to make a deep *impression*, to *carve*. A brutal example of this would be the making of a deep branding impression on the skin of a slave and so branding him or her, declaring "I own you." Or a Nazi soldier may pin a Star of David on the chest of a Jewish person to signify a target that must be burnt.

I now want to take these two, *line* and *character*, together. The cut into a line introduces a rupture in the identity of a people, creating a potential gap in their world. The branding, which once existed in the original mandate of slavery, can now change from one hand to another. A reversal of agency preserves the poisonous history. Horizonal [sic] with the words "broken line" and "character" are two terms used by the French psychoanalyst Jean Laplanche: "intromission" and "implantation." He uses those terms with respect to individual pathological formations. However, they will serve my description of shared injury to and branding of a people. Laplanche (1999) writes that "implantation is a process which is common, every day, normal or neurotic" (p. 136). But it has a virulent variant, and that is the one I wish to invoke here. Laplanche continues:

> Beside it [that is, apart from the normal or neurotic], as its violent variant, a place must be given to *intromission*. While implantation allows the individual to take things up actively, at once translating and repressing, one must try to conceive of a process which blocks this, short-circuits the differentiation of the agencies in the process of their formation, and puts into the interior an element resistant to all metabolization.
>
> (p. 136, italics in original)

According to Laplanche, then, *implantation* allows the injured party to actively take things up as well as to attempt to translate or repress the injury. *Intromission*, however, *forecloses translation or transformation.* Intromission renders the injury resistant to change. His words are worth echoing again and again: *intromission short-circuits differentiation and "puts into the interior an element resistant to all metabolization."* Referring to the body and its skin-envelope as well as the orifices of the body as metaphor, Laplanche writes: "*Intromission relates principally to anality and orality. Implantation refers, rather, to the surface of the body as* a whole, its perceptive periphery" (p. 137, emphasis added). I imagine from Laplanche's distinction that the skin remembers when it is broken into (implantation). This is true whether the breaking in has been in the form of a subject seeing and/or remembering a massacre of a people, in identi-fication, or in the form of a subject concretely and actively receiving pain from torture.

Forced intromission is a means of torture and shaming. Sodomy (intro-mission via anality) is known by perpetrators of ethnic violence as the most extreme shaming strategy. White New York City policemen forcibly inserting a broomstick into a black man's anus and mouth speaks amply to this issue of intromission as a shaming strategy. We can, of course, add intromission via genitality to the repertoire of shaming devices when per-petrators of ethnic violence rape the mothers, wives, and daughters of the enemy. In Laplanche's language, these strategies of forced intromission cause injuries that are not easily metabolized.

Under the rubric of *transgenerational haunting* I have evoked else-where (see Apprey, 1996) Carolivia Herron's (1991) description of generations of African Americans suffering the vicissitudes of transgen-erational trauma.

I shall summarize:

1   The females shall be raped by slave masters; the males shall be mur-dered by slave masters.
2   The males who are not murdered shall be sold away.
3   The males who are neither murdered nor sold away shall marry females who are not murdered or sold away.
4   In marriage, enslaved males and former slaves shall have revenge over females perceived to have consented to the destruction of males.
5   Women and daughters shall therefore be raped over and over again by enslaved men or former slaves.

In this sequence, three appropriative and appositional shifts and transfers occur:

1   the historical presentation of rape and murder in the first instance;
2   appropriation by an ethnic group of a transgressor's cruelty to serve a secondary purpose of revenge;

3   ossification of a structure of experience that says that victims may heap cruelty originating with external transgressors onto their own kind.

In transgenerational haunting, then, a contemporary generation is unwittingly possessed by an earlier generation. The possession preserves history, but in a poisonous, unmetabolized version. The sequence can be conceptualized as follows:

1   concrete staging;
2   doubling;
3   reactivation of sedimented historical grievances;
4   replay;
5   extension to serve contemporary purposes.

This transformation starts the process of *losing sight of one's historical enemies*.

Last, under the rubric of *figure*, we may think of disfiguring the Other. The torturer degrades and disfigures his object. The colonizer reduces a human being's status from a citizen to a non-person. The slave owner in the American South reduces a human being to, let us say, 3/5 of a person. The merchant refigures an impersonal exchange of goods (*metaphor*) into the *perverse metonymy* of selling persons, as in slavery. Dehumanization, par excellence, subserves this rubric.

I have so far considered history that which is potentially reconstituted by groups in conflict. Sedimentations of historical grievances are reactivated and then extended by those who relive them to serve new and contemporary purposes. In observing and working with aggrieved people, we have an obligation to learn *the actual historical injury* and how it has been mentalized and extended. When observing a people operating with a mandate to extinguish or enslave an Other group, we have the obligation to understand the historical motivation behind these acts of aggression.

Knowing the archaic mandate or errand will indicate how the aggrieved group has stored its historical memory. We need to know what the aggrieved group has stored in the imaginary space of a broken line. We need to know what reversals of agency have taken place. We need to know how harming their current target contributes to losing sight of their original enemy. We need to know the many ways in which grappling with a traumatic history has been deferred and the ways that this deferral contributes to the aggrieved group itself remaining disfigured, dehumanized, and traumatized as a people. Let us not forget self-contempt in some cases where identification with the aggressor keeps a traumatized person from claiming well-earned successes.

From the transgressor's end, we need to ask how the transgressor group stores its cultural memory. Owing to space limitations, I shall only list here and elaborate in subsequent work what I consider its central strategies:

1   the power to define socioeconomic, political, and even psychological issues in a community;
2   the power to write history and to publish according to the claims of the group that has greater power;
3   the power to disseminate that history;
4   the power to define how that history is taught in schools.

When, for example, American children are taught only US history from 1800 onward, a psychological statement is made to the children: that they may obliterate prior African and European history and define themselves in terms of the contemporary power relations between minority and majority groups. Therefore, in the work of conflict resolution, it is crucial to grasp the determinants and vicissitudes of ways that cultural memory from history is stored. During the conflict resolution process feuding parties are given opportunities to engage in an ongoing process where history can be staged, relived, and worked through. See the chapter "Containing the Uncontainable" in this book.

V. Praxis

What do injured communities put into the residual wound? How may they suture a ruptured history? How do they fill an absence? Appropriating the language of the French phenomenologist Maurice Merleau-Ponty (1983), I would say that the behaviors utilized by injured ethnic groups to fill the gap and suture the wound may be described as: (1) *syncretic,* (2) *symbolic,* and (3) *amovable.*

In *syncretic* behavior, the structure of experience is concrete and is embedded very tightly into the conditions of materiality. Tell an ape that this is a chair to sit on; the ape will most likely use the chair as a chair. Here, the structure of experience is very tightly immersed in the concrete conditions of materiality so that the signification chair as chair is the only expected one.

The structure of experience in *symbolic* behavior suggests that the behavior can be lifted from the conditions of concrete materiality and described *independently so that a symbol is both a thing and other than itself.* So, if you tell me that a chair is for me to sit on, I might add other and multiple functions. I can sit on it. In addition, I can hang my coat on the backrest. If this were a glass building and there were a fire, I could pick up that same chair, smash a window, and get out of the room.

In *amovable* behavior, there emerges an inchoate fantasy life in addition to some degree of symbolic differentiation. An adult may remember little from childhood while a phantom of a gloating cynical parent occupies his or her inner world. This phantom seems fixed in place. Efforts at change are not sustained. Change is frowned upon, or enacted with tremendous difficulty. Comparably, for the ancestors of once colonized or enslaved African Americans, the phantom may appear as an internal assassin that looks at his or her efforts at progress with *contempt.*

Why these three categories? The syncretic tells us about incest, murder, direct boundary violations, and other concretely staged acts of grievance or expressions of human desire. For example, "I saved her life, I can sleep with her." One may ask what saving a young woman's life has to do with sexual molestation. Such a syncretic juxtaposition of two unrelated issues can fill the wound of an absence. The immaturity of the adult is concretely injected into the immaturity of the wounded child. The adult believes the lie that saving a life has something to do with being granted sexual privilege. He believes that saving a life brings with it the right to damage a life. He acts as though a devastating past can be rightfully transposed from inside to outside, that devastation in his own history offers a sufficient account for his causing devastating, long-lasting injury to a girl, a daughter, a woman.

In this situation, a present-day African American man, to be described, houses ancestral figures who are in constant destructive conversations and internal war: the *ghosts* of a slave master turned rapist, a slave who is raped, tortured, or killed. In the words of Parveen Adams (1996), a British psychoanalytic scholar on sexual differences, "inside and outside rely on a certain coincidence rather than an opposition" (p. 148). For her the terms inside and outside are radically implied in each other. She adds:

"Within such reasoning, the subject, a space of interiority, establishes a relation with the world, a space of exteriority which consists in just the right amount of internalization and externalization for normality to exist and persist" (p. 149). For her, the interior and exterior, linked but separate, have a "preordained isomorphism" (p. 149) where the two spaces are invariably already there, already made for each other, yoked and yet separate. In a word, and in my formulation, interior and exterior are for the subject who is tied to a syncretic way of behaving, *consciousness syntonic*. We would normally say ego syntonic in psychoanalysis. I hold that *the ghost, the host, and the guest are now one agent who is today urgently striving to repeat historical injury, choosing an inappropriate object to attack during the repetition and haphazardly repeating the errand toward extinction or haphazardly re-creating a wayward child.*

In the case of amovable behavior, there is a new signification where there are *partial shifts* with particular meanings. For example, a woman whose conduct-disordered child I successfully treated said to me, "You treated my child and I thank you. I am not your patient. I will see a psychiatrist for medication for my Tourette's syndrome." Six months later, I heard on the radio that she had been dismissed by her school for harassing her students by taping their mouths when she felt that they talked too much. Some of the ramifications of this case will be discussed later, as part of my consideration of "the amovable." Now, instead of our dealing with and treating the consequences of incest by her father, the whole community was dealing with who causes injury to whom, what constitutes harassment, and what happens when a Black tenured college professor is on trial in an institution dominated by Whites in powerful positions.

Here the slave master has been internalized as an internal saboteur, an internal assassin. This internalized figure kills off the subject's will to recovery and constantly and cynically gloats at the subject's failures. The phantom of an assassin reigns in this domain. Any potential success alternates with self-destructive activity. The phantom demands that extinction in one form or another be avidly pursued. The phantom is merciless in demanding a destruction that is already mandated. The subject is left to choose her form of self-destruction.

In contrast, *symbolic behaviors have given the internal assassin a decent burial, knowing that the phantom is part of the self and cognizant that the ghost may return if one is not vigilant or resilient.* Adams might suggest here that the internal object of the assassin may be "emptied out."

To the notion of "emptied out" I would prefer the notion that the destructive agency of the internal assassin is *deferred* or *suspended* without any suggestion that the emptying out is final.

These three categories—syncretic, amovable, and symbolic—are phenomenological. They are a starting point and are not meant to be exhaustive or frozen into fixed compartments. After all, and as you will see over and over again in this book, there is no behavior that never descends below the symbolic level and no behavior that never rises above the syncretic level.

Following are some clinical vignettes intended to illuminate the distinctions: syncretic, amovable, and symbolic.

The Syncretic: The Perpetrator of Incest Who Juxtaposes Two Dissonant Causes

Returning to the "transgressor" who says, "I saved her life when she was a child and so I felt I could sleep with her," let us examine how the syncretic may move to the amovable. A horrified clinician may focus on the primitive thinking associated with this rationalization of incest. A morally outraged clinician might focus on the status of incest as crime. A disciplined phenomenologist, however, no less moral or ethical, will be able to read a multiplicity of meanings in this act of incest. For example, capturing the many sides of the subject's naive and syncretic thought, the phenomenologically disciplined clinician might be able to hear the following:

> Many years ago, I was terrified that she would die. In fact, I already gave her up for dead. It dawned on me that I could resuscitate her. I did, and fortunately she lived. She was six years old at the time. Eight years later, when she was fourteen, *I just did it, not thinking anything about it.* Now, when I look back, it does not seem right.

A time warp collapsed two time frames of the time of saving her life and the time of *incest* into a *syncretic* structure of behavior.

The 14-year-old would soon have three more children with her much older brother-in-law and psychological father. Then and as an adult, she was haunted by profound superego anxiety in an *amovable* structure of experience. It was up to her teenage daughter, whom I subsequently treated, to overturn the received historical injury in a *symbolic* way so that she could live with relative freedom.

The Amovable: Tiger, Aged Fourteen

Tiger is an African American boy whose mother brought him to treatment because he tried on more than one occasion to jump out of moving school bus.

> *Throughout her latency years, Tiger's mother was sexually abused, sodomized by her father, a minister of religion, in the basement of his church.*

When Tiger's mother married and conceived him, she dreamt in the third trimester that a Buddha figure wanted her to name him "Tiger." He would become a "tiger." In the brief period of treatment (three months), his main symptoms all involved *boundary violations*: running his bicycle into a person, breaking into an ATM, taking his mother's car and running into a bicyclist. Residential treatment was clearly called for. This was a successful placement. He lettered in three sports and won a scholarship to a four-year college.

After placing Tiger in a residential school, I asked the mother to consider treatment for herself. She refused. Two years after she refused treatment from me, Tiger died in a bungee-jumping accident.

Residential treatment took care of the behavioral problems but not the transgenerational transmission of destructive aggression. That toxic errand would remain *unspoken*. Witness the acting out, the remembering in action by the mother when as a school teacher *she would tape the mouths of children she felt talked too much*, the action that let to her public humiliation and ouster from her tenured position.

Tiger and his mother each suffered from the destructive aspects of unmetabolized histories. In each of them, and in the dyad formed by the two of them, there was a conjunction between *identification with the damaged parts of the internal parents and transgenerational haunting*. In both mother and son, one can sense the presence of the sexually abusing previous generation; this presence persists across generations while actually blocking the generative activity of generations. Instead of movement from one generation to the next, generations are crossed with each other, with disastrous consequences; his premature death and her humiliation. The efforts at *mentalization* by these patients are insufficient. The excessive burden of external transgressions seems to actually occupy their minds, like a living presence. The result leaves them degraded, humiliated, and haunted, in a state of perpetual devastation.

The Amovable: A Gruesome Haunt Outside the African American Community

I mentioned at the onset that these cases are not particular to the African American community.

A nine-year-old White American girl, Blanche, was treated by a psychologist who sought my help with the case. I supervised the case about 30 years ago when Blanche was hospitalized in Vienna, Virginia. She had been referred for in-patient treatment by a community mental health center where she had been in treatment for some 14 months along with her sister, three years younger, whom we shall call Lucinda. During this period of treatment, she was also prepared by a forensic team to testify against her biological mother and her boyfriend for child abuse. An abuse investigation had been initiated because Lucinda exhibited unusual sexual behavior in kindergarten, where she kept drawing explicit sexual pictures and exposing herself. The hearing resulted in the mother's acquittal because the girls could not testify publicly in court against her. They froze every time the opportunity to testify came. However, in videotaped testimonies, Blanche described rituals resembling satanic worship. She described robes, candles, and a noose hanging from the ceiling to warn the children not to talk about what they had seen. At the witch coven, *they drank blood* and consumed body parts, including the heart and liver of the dead. Shortly after the two girls were removed from their mother and placed in a foster home, Lucinda became hysterical when Blanche cut her finger, screaming that Blanche was not to put blood on her. Neither Blanche nor Lucinda would eat red meat at first, and they would not eat chicken off the bone because of its resemblance to body parts. In addition, Lucinda had phobic reactions to books; she feared that certain words and numbers could harm her. Further investigation by the police revealed that Blanche was being prepared to sacrifice Lucinda in order to inherit her special position as head of the witch coven.

Great-grandmother had passed on the role of head of the coven to grandmother, who had passed it on to Blanche's mother. In order to

*inherit that special role and robe, Blanche was to show unflinching
courage and kill Lucinda.*

Thankfully, this process was disrupted by the police, who had inadvertently learned about this sacrifice during their investigation of a missing eight-year-old girl who had disappeared on her way home from school.

Events that precipitated Blanche's referral included complaints by her foster brother that she had engaged in oral sex with the family dog, and, in addition, Blanche and Lucinda engaged in oral and genital stimulation every night. Upon referral, the staff wrote that *"Blanche had identified with the aggressor and had internalized negative devil image* [sic]" of herself.

In child psychotherapy Blanche expressed ambivalence about returning to her mother. She wanted to return home and yet was petrified to do so. She struggled with guilt about the killings in which she had participated. However, there was little remorse associated with her demonstrations of destructive aggression against her sister and foster brother.

Much of this successful treatment revolved around Blanche's effort to identify with her therapist as a new object while she reworked the mental representation of her internal parents. Details of this case are published elsewhere (see Kelly & Apprey, 1990).

The Symbolic: Going on an Unconscious Errand to Symbolically Restore a Dead Son to One's Parents

The symbolic type is quite unlike the amovable and the syncretic. It is like all compromise formations and post-structural pathological formulations. Arlanda is an African American female district court judge who came to see me because of what she described as longstanding anxiety related to the task of adjudicating cases.

After three months of once weekly psychotherapy, it dawned on her that she had all her adult life been "trying to put together the gentle and forceful sides" of her. She was trying to mend the component instinctual trends of masculinity and femininity, passivity and activity, and the ambivalence that went along with them.

Further exploration made her aware that she was troubled by her mother's unresolved mourning over the death of her first child, a son. She unconsciously wished to assuage her mother's grief. To do that, she would become the son her mother had lost. Choosing a male-dominated career, she insisted, served that illusion. The illusion was also useful in her relation to her father. He had two daughters, including her, and by becoming a judge, she might also become the son he never had.

Discovery of these issues made her aware that these unmended internal conflicts were part of the anxiety-provoking interethnic issues and power relations that she faced at work. She had previously been able to rationalize her anxiety as being solely related to racism. The rest of the treatment enabled her to renegotiate the capacity to entertain a multiplicity of skills and competencies that could more freely be experienced in different ways and at different times without the burden of having to describe those activities as masculine or feminine, passive or active.

VI. Differentiating Toxic Errands

The participants in each of these cases are on unconscious errands. Those on syncretic and amovable errands are on patently destructive paths. Those on symbolic errands are looking for, more or less, nondestructive forms of transformation. The symbolic errand tends to mimic the usual compromise formations that lead to post-structural or neurotic pathological formations or dysfunctions and may not necessarily lead to destruction.

The phenomenological categories of syncretic, amovable, and symbolic are useful in theorizing clinical work aimed at fostering emancipation from transgenerational haunting in individual work.

When we work with groups such as fractured communities in interethnic conflict, issues of communal memory and identification become privileged, and they become attached to modes of psychical transfer of destructive aggression across generations (Apprey, 2014). In the project of transformation in interethnic disputes, however, the sense of self changes. One enters an ethnic tent (Volkan, 1992), and transgenerational errands are transmitted across generations by leaders who embody a collective sense of self. In any case, some basic assumptions guide this sense of self that needs to be sustained as cohesive.

Corollary 1: In the field of conflict resolution, any conception of the Other as fixed or absolute dangerously lends itself to the readiness to dehumanize the Other.

Corollary 2: The facile notion that "we are one blood" is not a helpful solution because it poses a threat to a much needed sense of self-stability and differentiation. This imperative can take different forms, from flag waving to extinction of the Other.

Corollary 3: Of even greater threat to participant groups in conflict is any notion of the self as changing or relative because a precipitous readiness to change poses a threat to a group's identity.

Self as agency is therefore an approximation; the Other as absolute is a misnomer. When Self and Other engage in a process of resolution of a conflict, a new opportunity opens up. Optimally, this fosters a measured exchange of representations of Self and Other. When the process is well modulated by facilitators, four waystations typically emerge: (1) polarization: each side defines itself while demonizing the Other; (2) differentiation: each side recognizes the multiplicity of positions in each separate group; (3) crossing of mental borders: each side engages the Other in a metaphor-driven and meaningful dialogue, replacing old concrete passions with a new order of designations, propelled by an ethic of responsibility; and (4) ethical statements become grounded when participant groups join forces to create concrete and mutually beneficial projects.

VII. In Place of a Conclusion: Making Explicit Some Basic Assumptions Behind Ethnic Hatred, Reactivation of Violence, and Repair of Transgenerational Trauma

In the realm of ethnic violence, hatred, and conflict, ethnic groups operate with various degrees of awareness of their conception that "blood must not mix." As a result, they struggle with a tension between the defensive use of this conception of difference/identity and an adaptive use of it. When it is *defensive*, it is used to obviate the anxiety of contamination by an Other group. They may therefore proceed to diminish, humiliate, or kill the Other. When it is adaptive, it may be used for the purposes of self-definition of the group that fears contamination or destruction to define itself and its needs.

In working with individuals so traumatized, clinicians must grasp through transference and extra transference processes (1) sedimentations of historical grievances that have faded away, (2) forms of reactivation of those hitherto repressed matters, and (3) supplementations or extensions of that which has been recalled into the transference to serve a motivational purpose of revenge against a previous wrong or some other form of hatred.

The sedimentation, reactivation, and motivational extension operates as an unconscious *errand*. This errand is urgently driven by the mandate of history, such as "be nothing, die, or be bound to a transgressor." In other words, one's life must not be one's own. The person who is the object of hatred, then, may embrace the injection of destructive aggression and carry out the mandate to die. On the other hand, the person who is the object of hatred can create a new ethic of responsibility that says, "I must transform the received hatred."

In the case of groups that have been injured, there is invariably a pooled communal memory that also has undergone sedimentation and as such can be reactivated and extended to seek new and motivational purposes. Work with such groups requires careful observation and a systematic evolution of a group process that typically accommodates the following: (1) polarization between two feuding factions; (2) paradox and multiplicity between each faction; (3) the crossing of mental borders between the two groups that hate each other; and (4) the establishment of an ethic of responsibility where they may agree that they might not like each other, but at least they can trade together and work together for the common good of all. If such a fourfold process is not negotiated between the warring factions, any precipitous attempt to find common ground might be perceived as "incest" and thus compromise the project of collaboration.

In both individual and group projects of self-extinction, there is an identification with the damaged part of the internal parents and/or transgressor. Such a cynical internal transgressor gloats at the failure of the transgressed individual or group and constantly teases them with new ways of self-destruction. In unsuccessful cases it becomes a matter of picking one's own psychological poison.

Such psychological toxins, as it were, can be stored in syncretic, amovable, or symbolic ways. When the storage is syncretic, clinicians must look out for constructed justifications by the transgressed individual to perpetrate and justify further injury on others. When the storage is amovable, the phantom keeps eluding the transgressor and injured persons alike, wreaking havoc, often causing death to oneself and/or to others.

When the storage is symbolic, we have the usual neurotic compromise formations and/or pathological formulations that lend themselves more easily to treatment than their syncretic or amovable counterparts of storage.

My view of transgenerational trauma, fueled by ethnic violence and repair, brings together drive theory and a transgenerational object relations theory by radicalizing a developmental history of instinctual goals in the following way. This will serve as my refrain throughout the book.

In dialoguing with drive theory, we may no longer claim that the source of an instinctual impulse is the subject's body alone; rather, the source of an instinct can also be from an anterior (m)other or even multiple agents. We can no longer claim that an instinctual drive operates exclusively with urgency; rather, an instinct can be both urgent and deferred through a deceptively dormant intercession between generations. We can no longer state that an instinct's singular aim is to seek satisfaction of libidinal or aggressive ends through an active or passive avenue; rather, those instinctual aims can be collapsed into one another and compromised, as when a subject accepts an infanticidal project from another only to contest it and/or transform it. We can no longer perceive an object that performs or participates in a subject's libidinal or aggressive aims as the object of desire, hostile dependence, and so on; rather, we must think of objects as though they were simultaneously potentially independent, potentially intermediary, as well as potentially a member in a series of linkages, as subjects in apposition, for example, across generations.

The marriage of concepts from drive theory and object relations theory allows us to see that (1) drive processes begin the activation of agency (doing to or poisoning) and that (2) human interaction becomes an epistemic place where the drama of human action takes place. Then (3) humans as agents enter the clinical space as a public place where change can be negotiated.

Seeing humans as caught up in the whirlwind of these noxious processes, I submit that the idea of "urgent/voluntary errands" allows us to face the fact of innate aggression and its urgent expression, on the one hand, and, on the other hand, we can also face our ethic of responsibility to find new and voluntary means of choosing our poison or transforming human and destructive aggression. Hope and responsibility occupy the second half of the notion of "urgent voluntary errands."

References

Adams, P. (1996). *The Emptiness of the Image: Psychoanalysis and Sexual Differences*. London & New York: Routledge.

Apprey, M. (1996). Broken lines, public memory, absent memory: Jewish and African Americans coming to terms with racism. *Mind and Human Interaction*, 7(3): 139–149.

Apprey, M. (1999). Reinventing the self in the face of received transgenerational hatred in the African American community. *Journal of Applied Psychoanalytic Studies*, 1(2): 131–143.

Apprey, M. (2014). "Containing the uncontainable." The return of the phantom and its reconfiguration in ethnonational conflict resolution. *The American Journal of Psychoanalysis*: 162–175.

Auden, W. H. (1954). On this island. In *The Major Parts: English and American*, ed. Charles M. Coffin, p. 541. New York: Harcourt Brace and World.

Hartmann, H. (1958). *The Ego and the Problem of Adaptation*. New York: International Universities Press.

Herron, C. (1991). *Forever Jonnie*. New York: Random House.

Husserl, E. (1929). *Cartesian Meditations: An Introduction to Phenomenology*. Translated by D. Cairus. The Hague: Martinus Nijhoff.

Iser, W. (1992). Staging as an anthropological category. *New Literary History*, 23(4): 877–888.

Kelly, M. M. & Apprey, M. (1990). Witchcraft as a source of psychic trauma. In *Clinical Studies and Their Translations*, ed. H. F. Stein & M. Apprey, pp. 62–103. Charlottesville, VA: University Press of Virginia.

Laclau, E. (1990). *New Reflections in the Revolution of Our Time*. London & New York: Verso.

Laplanche, J. (1999). *Essays on Otherness*. London & New York: Routledge.

Lotman, Y. & Uspensky, B. A. (1971). On the semiotic mechanism of culture. In *Critical Theory Since 1965*, eds. H. Adams & L. Searle, pp. 412–413. Tallahassee: Florida State University Press and University Presses of Florida.

Merleau-Ponty, M. (1983). *The Structure of Behavior*. Pittsburgh, PA: Duquesne University Press.

Miller, J. H. (1992). *Ariadne's Thread: Story Lines*. New Haven, CT: Yale University Press.

Volkan, V. D. (1992). Ethnonationalistic rituals: An introduction. *Mind and Human Interaction*, 4(1): 3–19.

Chapter 4

"Scripting" Inhabitations of Unwelcome Guests, Hosts, and Ghosts

Unpacking Elements That Constitute Transgenerational Haunting

1   *The most common phrase in the literature is that of the transgenerational transmission of trauma. In your own writing, you often use the phrase "<u>transgenerational haunting</u>." Since your choice of words is rarely casual, I am wondering what additional meaning you seek to convey through this phrase to the understanding of unconscious, transgenerational processes.*

Thank you, Bill, for asking for this clarification between "transgenerational transmission of trauma" and "*transgenerational haunting*." The word *trauma*, taught by Anna Freud when I was a student at the Hampstead Clinic, now the Anna Freud Centre, was at one time strictly limited to the *shattering of the ego* with *distortion of ego functions as a consequence*. The more recent plastic use of the term trauma to include multiple and painful or psychologically disorganizing consequences of a temporary nature, therefore, misses what structural damage trauma specifically inflicts on the ego and its executive functions for a subject. On the other hand, *transgenerational haunting speaks* to a sequence of happenings: (1) an injection, an implantation, of an unmetabolized unconscious mandate by a parent or by an ancestral figure; an aggressive interiorization that is (2) subsequently *suspended inside the psyche* (3) until it shall have found a suitable object of exteriorization. One may say that there are suitable alternative terms like identification, projective identification, intrusive identification, incorporation, identification with the aggressor, and so on. All these nomenclatures are, to use the phenomenological term, horizonal [sic], but they are not interchangeable; horizonal in terms of proximity but not identical. A haunt stays within a descriptive and yet powerful phenomenological framework that keeps the process alive.

DOI: 10.4324/9781003389026-5

Anthropologically, a haunt speaks to an appropriation of a *possession*, desirable or undesirable.

I recall from my catalogue of childhood memories in Ghana, West Africa, hearing more than one elder say of a child: "this child has been here before." In such circumstances, there may be a reference to *an ancestor who has returned and possesses an other [sic] body*. In French, the idea of a ghostly return has been preserved. A ghost is a "revenant"; one who returns. Nicholas Abraham, who wrote of the "phantom" as a meta-psychological construct, says in "Notes on the Phantom: A Complement to Freud's Metapsychology" (1975) that "The belief that the spirit of the dead can return to haunt the living exists as an accepted tenet or as a marginal conviction in all civilizations, ancient or modern" (p. 171). Then he eloquently adds a *motivation* for the return: "More often than not, the dead do not return to join the living but rather to lead them into some dreadful snare, entrapping them with disastrous consequences" (p. 171). Who are those that are destined to return, he ponders? "The dead who were shamed during their lifetime or those who took unspeakable secrets to their grave" (p. 171). Abraham is here using the word haunt to make a distinction between the quotidian existence of family secrets that need not necessarily feed the creation of a symptom and what we may now paraphrase as the *mystification of secrets*, that is, the lies families tell to conceal a secret for a defensive purpose in order to mitigate anxiety. In his account, the mystification of secrets subsequently feeds pathological formations.

I use the word "haunting" as part of the work of the clinical process of Nachträglichkeit that Freud *insufficiently* translated as deferred action. *A "haunt" fills in the gap between injection and deferral. In short, a subject has to store and suspend for some time during an incubation period an implant, as it were, before a deferral can take place.* This is a perfect time to bring in Eric Berne: "The most intricate part of *script analysis* in clinical practice is tracing back the influences of the grandparents" (1972, p. 288). I am grateful to you, Bill, for supplying this quote from Berne. A script has to have a source. Second, it has to be suspended for an incubation period before it can wreak havoc on its *host*. Third, the *unwelcome guest must change places with the host before the onward deferral can take place*. We can now be more precise: The most intricate part of script analysis is the tracing back to *an anterior source* the transfer of uncanny psychological presences from unwelcome ancestral guest(s) to the *colonized host*. Here, we are not looking for mechanisms but for motivation for the injection:

motivation for the hosting in the face of surrender. Now the injection is fixed and stable; a script. Now it is *structured* and *predictable*. Treatment must now focus on what can be fostered to emerge in the room, into the transference, where that which has been deferred, and scripted for transfer, can become resubjectivized in the present unconscious of the patient.

2   *You trained in both child and adult psychoanalysis within relatively classical models. Your attention to transgenerational processes has been a part of your writing and work from very early on. How did you first come to recognize* <u>*the centrality of transgenerational haunting?*</u> *How has it shaped your work as an analyst?*

How then did I come to recognize the centrality of transgenerational haunting?

I have never seen transgenerational haunting and subsequent trans-mission(s) as a departure from Freud's classical models. Rather, I see transgenerational haunting as something that has always been there, almost invariably, already in the patient's history. How a clinician understands human development and uses that fund of knowledge to take a history of a new patient is central to transgenerational inquiry. We can elaborate on this shortly with vignettes from clinical material. Before then, let us ask some questions that emerge *when two human subjects court each other* for a meaningful relationship before children enter into that potentially stable relationship and develop.

Multiple traditions of psychoanalysis and psychology, in general, think of stages of human development after birth, usually from zero to three. Let us, then, consider starting with conscious and unconscious motivations for *recruiting each other* for marriage. Along the way, let us explore the responses of each family to each partner before a marriage takes place. When children are considered or not before or after marriage, what would become the manifest or latent function the children would come to serve for their parents? What is the history of the link between the parents; how much do they love and care for each other in the eyes of the child?

When, additionally—and this is pivotal—the history of the three trimes-ters of pregnancy are considered in a case, we want to know what *psychi-cal* experience of *fusion* correlates with the *physical* template of biological *fusion* in the first trimester. After kicking begins in the second trimester, we want to know what psychical experiences of *differentiation* correlate with the biological template. In the third trimester, we want to grasp what psychical experiences of *separation* correlate with the physical separation. When *the physical delivery* of the infant from its mother occurs, what *psychical delivery of the young mother from her own mother* occurs?

When we give up the phantasy that the stork brought the child, when we take the psychology of pregnancy into our accounts of human development, we can appreciate a young pre-psychotic mother's cry that she must not tell her mother she is pregnant because her mother would kill her, or the news of the pregnancy would kill her mother. I have learned so much from variations of three-generational psychological warfare, as it were, in puerperal psychosis and severe cases of post-natal depression. This phenomenon of being *taken over* by a persecutory internal object, an inside parent, is not unique to puerperal psychosis or severe post-natal depressions. We see it in recovering anorexics or bulimics who conceive, carry, and then deliver a baby to term. Although these extreme conditions appear to be exceptions to the psychology of pregnancy and delivery, all these conditions I have just mentioned, nevertheless, tell us something urgent about taking in hostile internal presences that shape our lives before we are equipped to negotiate internal fields of reference to the outside and external fields of reference to the inside.

Maurice Merleau-Ponty once said, and I am paraphrasing it, human beings teach us so much with their exceptions. An exception freezes that which looks like an exception long enough for the rest of us to see ourselves in that so-called exceptional phenomenon. Psychoanalytically, *early and deep are synonymous*, and therefore *we get to see inchoate forms of lived experience* when we do early infant observations and/or when we work with psychotic and near-psychotic parents of infants. Put these two ideas together: one about exceptions, the other about early and deep, and you can appreciate that seemingly "extraordinary" persecutory anxiety a regressed newborn mother might feel that if her mother visits after the birth of her infant her mother would eat her newborn baby. Cannibalistic anxieties are exceptional, to be sure, in non-clinical spheres of life, and yet, in clinical narratives, the ordinary and extraordinary alternate.

Linking Freud's structural theory to the idea of three generations, we get the following: (1) the id bespeaks the fullness of the fleshly illusion of "paradise" of the mother-infant relationship, (2) the superego as the prohibition of the potentially incestuous tie and the symbolization of the prohibition into aim and direction in life, and (3) the ego as *the mother's identification with her mother*. I would further clarify the mother's relationship to her mother as the building up of the ego in the following way: the mother as auxiliary ego to her child to whom she is *physically linked* must simultaneously work through the *psychical connections* to her own mother. The representation of that psychical connection informs what she consciously or unconsciously proceeds to do with her child. She does so with various degrees of identification and disidentification *with her mother*.

This is a very long way to answer your question about how I came to understand transgenerational transmission within a Freudian framework. *One* of the ways I came to understand transgenerational transmission, then, was through studying disturbed and at-risk mothers in pregnancy and childbirth. Baldly, *we cannot understand transgenerational transmission without understanding a mother's tie to her mother and, subsequently, how a newborn mother "empties out" the contents of her unmetabolized ego into the ego of her child. It is this fragile tie between the mother as an auxiliary ego and her tie to the inchoate ego of the child that led Freud (1916) to say that the early ego is not a master in its own house*. It is subject to implantation (Laplanche, 1999). Freud's use and translation of the German word *"Zartlichkeit"* as "affection" must in this context be translated as a *"porous tenderness."* Into this porous and tender world, an inchoate ego that is not a master in its own house must sort through and select, over time, ancestral voices, demands, prescriptions, and constraints.

A clinical vignette would help to elaborate this *emptying out into a porous, tender, and affectionate place.*

> Jerome is a four-year-old African American boy. He is brought to a university child and family clinic by his parents at the insistence of his pre-school teacher who sees him biting, pushing, and punching other children *instead of speaking out* what he desires. *He is four and still has no speech.* He is without any clear words. *Like an infant, he is without speech; he babbles.* In his first meeting with a resident, a young psychiatrist in training, he puts his hands between the buttons of the shirt of his diagnostician and rubs his little hands against the chest of this new person he has only just met. The resident is intrigued. He ponders what this insertion of hands into an unfamiliar place means. The attending psychiatrist and a clinical team, who are watching this first interview behind a mirror for training purposes, are horrified. They insist that the resident report the case to the local social

services for investigation of possible child abuse. The resident is now horrified by a recommendation he deems a premature judgement and comes to see me for supervision. Because he has not even taken a history, I invite the parents to come and provide a history. This following is what is in the history. To preserve the vividness of the history, let us speak in the present tense for a while. Jerome's father has *a father* who is so *physically violent* that Jerome's paternal grandmother takes all his children into her house to raise them across the street. Jerome's mother has *a father* who is *both physically and sexually violent.* He insists on forcing himself on his daughters. He commits *incest with the oldest daughter.* She succumbs. In the incestuous father's mind, *the second daughter must follow* suit. *She refuses him. He kills her* and is now in jail. *Jerome's mother*, one of the younger daughters, *is spared.*

When Jerome's parents grow up and find each other they predetermine that *no violence must occur in their home.* They are *perfect recruits* for each other. They consciously do not want to see a repeat return of the violence they themselves once encountered in their own turn as parents. They have recruited each other to raise a child in *a new and perfectly non-violent home.* However, they are about to be ambushed. How? Jerome starts life with a serious case of colic. He is terribly difficult to hold and comfort. They declare that *he must not hurt or be hurt.* He must not want. They take him into their marital bed and he sleeps there until the day his parents come to see me four years later. What must I do with this situation? I insist he must stay in his own bed, and the next day, I would like to see them in order to complete taking their family history and the child's developmental history. Mother protests that he cannot sleep alone. Nevertheless, and to her utmost surprise, *he sleeps in his bed throughout the night and nothing untoward happens.* She comes to see me the next morning with her hair done, smiling happily, and very pleased with herself and her son.

Into that loving embrace of his mother, into that tender and porous matrix, an inchoate, unformed infantile ego has ingested the unmetabolized toxins *through constraints and prescriptions* of what to do and what not to do. Memories of violent fathers persist. They cannot shake off those violent and incestuous memories. Here is the ambush. Thinking they are trying to avert history, they unwittingly force an identification between a combined imago of two grandfathers and Jerome. They do not know that an extreme desire to disidentify that representation of violent and incestuous grandparents is but the surest way to pass on what is consciously rejected. They do not know that two *extreme opposites*, not any ordinary reaction formations or over-compensation, are but the same behavior; only one side thoroughly conceals the other. They therefore unwittingly ensure the return of a combined, violent and/or incestuous grandfather who respects no boundaries. I supervise the child psychotherapy case of the resident psychiatrist. I treat the parents. They must now reformulate what their new mission as a couple must be and can become. *The child can now speak his needs* and can start kindergarten and no longer serve as the host of a murderer and possibly become the murderer himself. He grew up eventually, I am happy to attest, as himself!

3   *Central in your clinical approach to transgenerational transmission is what you describe as the unconscious translation of the events of history to a sense of history (2006). To that end, you outline a process of the past emerging in the present from "sedimentation" to "reactivation," and finally "intentionality." Can you provide our readers with a brief description of this process emphasizing the emergence of reactivation of transgenerational demands through the transference relationship, expressing both transferential demands and wishes?*

How then does a subject go from *the events of history* to *a sense of history?* First, and starting from the ground up, a series of *nodal points* appear in the history. They fade away like sediments into the base, as it were. The *sedimentations of history* will await resonance of contemporary material that Freud termed "identity of perception" in Chapter 7 of his *Interpretation of Dreams* (1900). Second, there is *reactivation*, where a subject will select elements from the sedimentations and mentalize them. We are now in the realm of a personal ideographic story; a personal psychology, a representation of that which has now been awakened and remembered. Third, that which shall have been awakened can now serve a new purpose; an *intentional emancipatory project that through the transference will become an ethical basis for a resubjectivization, further away from the original haunt,* as it were. Here, in the transference, a patient will make a plea, a demand, a request, and nudge the clinician in order to both *repeat* and to *reconfigure*. A *re-enactment would only serve as a demand for a clinician to be a witness that she was once harmed.* I acknowledge my potential role as a witness, but I am underwhelmed. *We must move forward with the project of emancipation; a process that requires a resubjectivization that would in turn fuel a sublimation potential as we move forward with processes of transformation.*

Let us consider, then, the vignette of one case that had an unfavorable outcome and contrast it with a case that came to a successful and planned termination. These two fragments will tell us the difference between *enactments as "dead ends"* and *the capacity to reconfigure and resubjectivize in the process of transformation.*

In favorable circumstances, I am able to hear a narrative revealed over time. This narrative has two parts: *a larger configurational narrative* composed of multiple, derivative, and *episodic pieces* that will in the end constitute a whole. In unfavorable circumstances, a family might reject treatment only to reenact the transgenerational narrative *without transformation of the psychological toxin*, as it were.

Now a tragic fragment.

Partha is an early adolescent child who is breaking into other people's spaces and causing potential harm to them: breaking out of a moving school bus, stealing his mother's bank debit card and using it to illicitly take her money, riding his bicycle into crowds and hitting a pedestrian, smoking marijuana, and so on and so forth. The school gives his mother the ultimatum to have the child treated or be expelled. When he is referred to me, I take a history. So let us go back in history. Mother as a latency child of 6 to 12 years of age is sexually molested by her father, a religious man, a practicing Baptist minister in his office in the basement of a church while he exotically burns incense until an aunt rescues her and removes her from the house and restores whatever developmental functions of the executive ego are possible after repeated, sexual, and traumatic attacks on a child's mind and body.

As a young adult in her 20s, as if she deserved to be punished, she marries a man who loves her and leaves her pregnant. In the third trimester, she dreams of a Buddha figure appearing in her dream. He mandates that her son's name shall be Partha, which he says means a "warrior." She obediently names him so.

After the assessment, I decide that he needs in-patient treatment first before I can treat him with psychotherapy. He goes to an in-patient unit that includes a residential school in its treatment regimen and prospers. He wins a wrestling scholarship to attend a community college and thrives. After two years, he is awarded an athletic scholarship to attend a prestigious four-year college. In the gap between completing a two-year community college and beginning a four-year college, he comes back home to visit his mother. On one Friday, he witnesses a robbery at a gas/petrol station. Now a good citizen, he is going to provide evidence to convict the criminal on Monday. On the Sunday before turning in state evidence, he goes bridge jumping, a poor man's version of bungee jumping. He witnesses a man drowning. He jumps from the bridge to save him. He hits his head against a rock in the river. He lifts his head once. He does not survive. The "warrior" dies.

This case is relevant because the mother and the schools were so busy celebrating his external successes that the psychological toxins were not overturned. *No resubjectivization took place either with the mother herself or with the son.* They rejected psychoanalytic advice at their peril. A year later, the mother, a teacher, is expelled for child abuse for taping the mouths of *students who talk too much.* Finally, she asks for treatment. I am able to offer it. She is able to receive it. Talking too much? What is too much to talk about? What must a child not talk about? To whom? Her own incest? To her mother? An aunt? Has she now lost sight of the original transgressor that crosses the generations by molestation? Just what must remain unspoken and taped away?

Now a second fragment of a case where there is optimal transformation.

In a second fragment, we have a case where there is resubjectivization of the received psychological toxin. *The script she carries with her is that a woman does not need a career.* A good woman takes care of her husband. She grows up to defy her grandmother, the planter of that precept of a script, by becoming a physician who does not practice after training. She obeys her grandmother by marrying a very wealthy man. The compromise: by marrying a wealthy man, she can afford not to practice as a physician. In the first year of analysis, an intrapsychic story is told through dreams, fantasies, and other forms of representation: a mothering figure of a pre-mammalian kind must drain everything from inside of her: from the digestive, reproductive, and urinary systems. She tortures me as no one has ever done. Every interpretation must be drained out.

By the end of the first year of treatment, it is palpable in the analysis that someone must die: which one of us would it be? At the very end of the first year, she stages my death: she brings me a gift for standing still and staying alive for her while she drains out of herself all her vital fluids. A castor oil plant that contains the poison, ricin, must be in my possession. I must plant it in my garden. At the end of the second year she stages her own death when she rejects my interpretations about the harm she inflicts on herself when she singlehandedly takes care of her husband's nine Arabian horses. In her fatigue, one of the horses falls on her and seriously breaks her hips. She survives. In the third year her history is represented in the transference as follows: "You must get a supervisor to help with my case. All analysts do that." She is certain. She has had three previous analysts and fired all three, she tells me. I am destined to be the fourth that she would fire if I do not get a supervisor. A pivotal dream after a torturous nine months of analysis comes to a head with a dream where she barely survives a rain/sand storm, a dream that I privately interpret to be the story of her birth but instead of saying so, I ask her to tell me the story of her birth. She is reluctant but does so. She tells me that she almost died.

A grandmother refuses to go to the hospital to stand behind her daughter for her delivery. "We deliver babies right here in the farm. We do not have to go to the hospital." The mother survives, but the grandbaby, my now-grown adult patient, almost dies, the umbilical cord wrapped around her neck three times. To repeat for emphasis, this history is represented in the transference as follows: "You must get a supervisor to help with my case. All analysts do that." She is certain. She has had three previous analysts and fired all three, she tells me. I am destined to be the fourth that she would fire if I do not get a supervisor. After my intervention and her *rediscovery* of the story of her birth that nearly ended in death she tells me that actually she fired a fourth psychoanalyst: "I told him that he looked like a Nazi before I fired him."

For three months, she would sleep like a baby, sometime holding her head as if to figure out the dimensions of her cranium and asking me to tell her the story of the mythical figure Narcissus in Ovid's *Metamorphosis*.

To sum up, a child is born. No one dies. She survives her birth. Her mother survives the delivery. Now, and for her, *there is an opportunity to work through her perilous beginnings.* For her mother, *a physical delivery of her baby is simultaneously a psychical delivery from her mother*, a project of three generations negotiating their emancipation from one another.

Grandma's errand to be nothing must be upended. I can now become a meaningful witness. The *urgent errand* to become nothing must be overturned. An *urgent enactment of self-erasure* must be replaced by *a voluntary errand that frees self from deadly ancestral mandates.* The transformation of potential death into life is now possible because by taking the negative transference of my patient by being steady and focusing on making meaning, I ensure her birth. She can now be psychically born. No enactment of an abortive situation takes place. Instead, there is a reformulation that a child with normal narcissism, normal needs, who can be parented, as it were, in treatment. A new world can now be resubjectivized. A new world emerged!

4   *Outside of the analytic dyad, in group and community relations, how do you see the unconscious expression and demands of the reactivation phase?*

In the external world, there is still resonance with the internal world, but not identity, between individual psychology and group psychology.

Whereas we can think of the *representational world in individual psychology*, we must now consider *communal memory in group psychology*.

Let us answer this question in two ways: first, a general conceptual sense using a psychoanalytic concept, and second, a specific point of conflict between two feuding communities.

Consider, for instance, the psychoanalytic concept of change of function over a time horizon of multiple generations.

Heinz Hartmann (1958) suggested that we humans do not come to terms with our environment anew in every generation. Rather, through the influence of traditions and the survival of previous creations of foregone eras, we appropriate from others a good many of our methods for solving problems.

Consequently, we live in other generations just as much as we live in our own.

After the fall of the Soviet Union, I was part of an interdisciplinary team doing ethno-national conflict resolution between Indigenous Estonians and Estonian Russians. One of the historical sites in Estonia is a cemetery with mass Jewish graves in Klooga. Klooga went through multiple phases in history: a concentration camp, a Soviet military site for deporting Estonians to Siberia, and today a site for NATO exercises.

Originally established in 1942 in German-occupied Estonia, the Klooga concentration camp functioned for two years as a forced labor sub-camp of the larger Vaivara concentration camp complex. However, the Germans exterminated 2000 Jewish prisoners in September 1944 before Russians could rescue the remainder. Subsequently, Klooga, no longer a concentration camp, became a Russian military camp. Here, anti-Soviet Estonians were gathered and exiled to Siberia. After the fall of the Soviet Union, Estonia became a member of NATO. Estonians transformed that same Klooga military field into a site for joint Baltic-NATO military exercises.

Shortly after Estonia *restored* its independence from the Soviet Union, an interdisciplinary group of psychoanalysts, historians, political scientists, and others were invited to mediate tensions between Indigenous Estonians and Estonian Russians.

The practice of ethno-national conflict resolution came in at this point. In small group processes, I documented the following four-part sequence.

In my account of the small group process in ethno-national conflict resolution (Apprey, 2014), the unpacking of *communal memory* begins with *polarization*. Accordingly, the communal memory of the Indigenous Estonians polarizes as follows: "We are Europeans. You Russians are Asians; some of you are even Mongolians. We will join the European Union and NATO and be with our Western European counterparts." The communal memory of the Estonian Russians was as follows: "You are our Serfs. We rescued you from the servitude of Serfdom. You betrayed us, the new Democrats from the Russian Federation. You should have worked with us instead of breaking away completely and treating Estonian Russians as non-citizens."

After polarization would come *irony and paradox*: In the communal memory of Estonians, we could hear something like this: "There are Estonians who fought with you Soviets against Nazis. There are Estonians who fought with Germans against Soviets. There are Estonians who did neither. Who is more Estonian?" On the side of Estonian Russians, "some of us Russians came to Estonia to *escape from religious persecution* during the time of the czar; some of us came because we *were sent* by the KGB; others came as *military personnel*. Now, who is to blame for Soviet crimes?"

After irony and paradox, further transformation of communal memory came as *the crossing of mental borders* with relative constraints like this and in their own words: "We have a long silence today. Perhaps the silence has come to serve as police so that we do not hurt each other." Or, instead of silence serving as a group superego, if I may so translate their behavior and words as restraint of hostilities, the two sides sometimes want to play: "You Russians want us to trust you. You know, when a man wants a woman to believe that he loves her, he must say it often enough so that she can believe him." The Russian response, "You Estonians call us the big fat elephant from *near abroad*. You are like rabbits. What will happen if an elephant mates with a rabbit? You get a mutant gene." These observations are so transparent that facilitators do not have to interpret them.

After a depressive and pregnant silence or after playfulness that serves as an infrastructure for a new representation of new possibilities, they would arrive at a fourth place—*a gesture of mediation*—where they would say something like this: "We may never totally trust each other, but at least we can trade together for our common good." This declaration serves as a new intentionality and respite from their hostilities.

Now, let us say something more about the question of two feuding factions remembering a collective history. I indicated earlier that Indigenous Estonians and Estonian Russians needed to sort out their differences after the breakdown of the Soviet Union.

One of the bones of contention was conflict between them as to where Estonia's boundaries ended and where those of the Russian Federation began. In 1920 Estonia had an extra 40 kilometers of land. Then the Soviet Union annexed that land and populated it with Russians. During the conflict resolution period, Estonians were torn. If they insisted on getting back their 40 kilometers of land, they would increase their Russian population, and it could become a significant electoral size. If, on the other hand, they forfeited the 40 kilometers of land, they would feel like a part of them was torn away from their body politic. The Estonian nationalists were clearly torn: Is Estonia's identity tied to land, especially land that is populated by an enemy? Is Estonia's identity one that is devoid of enemy inhabitants, albeit 40 kilometers smaller? The two sides had to work through this. Estonia eventually chose the latter—a smaller piece of territory devoid of enemy inhabitants.

5   *One of the most compelling ideas I find in your model of transgenerational hauntings is that of "urgent voluntary errands" that compel the enactment of transgenerational pressures within an individual and/or community. You argue that history itself has an urgency that cries out for repetition, recognition, and meaning and that the "urgently infused*

mandate" of a previous generation becomes appropriated in a later generation. What began as an urgent (dissociated?) projection and demand from one generation is taken up two generations later in a way that is seemingly now voluntary, even though it continues to carry all of the urgency of the crisis of the original generation. Could you address the question of time that is implicated in the demand to repeat?

We have touched on the developmental issue of pregnancy and childbirth as a three-generational process. In the process, we have alluded to a mother's identification with her mother as central to the process of transmission of unmetabolized unconscious matter that enters the field of a new-born mother and her infant. We know then that an infant's early ego is not a master in its own house and that it is subject to ancestral implantation. Zartlichkeit as *a fragile and porous template* has replaced Freud's Zartlichkeit as *affection*. Affection, albeit correct in a different context, is insufficient when we are describing the passing through of unmetabolized ancestral wishes; porous tenderness is more cogent in helping us to describe that which passes through this permeable mother-infant matrix. Similarly, the process of Nachträglichkeit that Freud translated as "deferred action" was insufficient. Jacques Lacan comes closer with his translation of deferred action as *"après-coup"* (Lacan, 1975). This term refers to *the circularity of enactments* in the deferral. In this circularity, a powerful and evocative transference scene is established in the treatment long after the creation of the original and historic genetic-developmental scene. In the throes of the transference, as I have indicated, historic scene I catches up with transference-laden scene II and hence *the après-coup*. Past and present are no longer linear but circular. A quick example. Let us revisit the previous patient who was told by her grandmother that a woman does not have to become a physician, so she must erase herself in order to exist for her husband. She worked through the following process with me. In the third year when she insisted that I get a supervisor to enable her analysis to succeed, she was establishing scene II. *Scene II was established in the treatment before scene I,* the history of a precarious birth was announced and came to catch up through de-repression, working through, the co-creation and mutual understanding of the meaning of our work. In her unconscious phantasy, a supervised analyst, like an expectant mother with her mother behind her, would ensure the psychological birth of an adult analysand. A grandmother's sturdy presence in her unconscious phantasy would ensure the safe and physical birth of a new-born child. In Lacan, there is then a circular temporality. We owe a debt of gratitude to Lacan for popularizing this circularity. In my own work, I observe a continuity of circles that bespeak *spiral causality*. In other words, there is circularity, to be sure, but there is a repeatable closing and opening of a circle as well as a repetitive change of form and function of the transference(s): a reconfiguration, as I interpret and detoxify the implantation. At this stage of the work, there is spirality of newer and newer transference manifestations in the form of working through. This spiral circularity is driven by two factors: (1) a mandated errand that has changed hands from an ancestral figure to an appropriating subject who will now take ownership and "pick one's own poison," so to speak, and (2) because there is a return to history where scene I catches up with scene II, a *pluperfect errand* is clinically established. In a past perfect tense, a human subject returns to itself. Translation: The phrase, "When I shall have done X," and by my own hand, is but *"I have been sent; only I do not know my sender, and I shall return home with the sense that I have done something for myself or for someone. That something has to be unpacked. That someone else for whom I carried out a bidding has to be disentangled from oneself."*

A subject that returns to itself is that which the Continental French philosopher Claude Romano (2009) named an "advenant." To be precise, sometimes when we think we have an active project, we have actually been sent on *an errand*. Here, an ancestral project, founded and foundered, placed or misplaced, long ago, still lingers, but in the hands of a new and suitable carrier. Past and present change places; subject and object change places. I, a subject, and once an object of another, *wander off* with a mandate, not of my own making but of a subject's appropriation. It is tempting to seek further clarity here. However, we cannot force any more clarity here because the process is initially opaque, unconscious, numinous, enigmatic, and decidedly obscured with *con-fusion* [sic]. Sometimes, *my errand makes me wander off*. Sometimes, *someone is in error, as in a mistake*, sometimes, *the moment I am named I have been sent off packing on a journey, on an errand and at a parent's or grandparent's bidding.* Whose errand is it? Whose bidding is it? Whose journey is it? *Who is held hostage on the errand? Who is mis-taken?* We humans, then, are often in an *ek-static* [sic] place as we stand outside of ourselves.

Vicissitudes of transference and countertransference processes come to our rescue to find our bearing and eventually anchor us as *we dramatize and transform the events of history into a represented sense of history in a new and public space* called *a clinical relationship*. Henceforth a new and potential errand of our own making and by our own hand and mind called *a sublimation* can be cultivated by the analysand.

References

Abraham, N. (1975). Notes on the phantom. In *The Shell and the Kernel*, Volume I. Chicago & London: The University of Chicago Press.

Apprey, M. (2014). Containing the uncontainable. *The American Journal of Psychoanalysis*, 74(2): 162–175.

Berne, E. (1972). *What Do You Say After You Say Hello? The Psychology of Human Destiny*. New York, NY: Grove Press.

Freud, S. (1900). The interpretation of dreams. In *Standard Edition*, Volume V. London: Hogarth Press and the Institute of Psychoanalysis.

Freud, S. (1916). A difficulty in the path of psychoanalysis. In *Standard Edition*, Volume 17. London: Hogarth Press and the Institute of Psychoanalysis.

Hartmann, H. (1958). *The Ego and the Problem of Adaptation*. New York: International University Press.

Lacan, J. (1975). *Seminaire XXII*. RSI, Ornicar: Bulletin périodique du champ Freudien.

Laplanche, J. (1999). *Essays on Otherness*. London & New York: Routledge.

Romano, C. (2009). *Event and World*. New York: Fordham University Press.

Chapter 5

Representing, Theorizing, and Reconfiguring the Concept of Transgenerational Haunting in Order to Facilitate Healing

AIZ SIEM VARTIEM VAID. ("Beyond these gates [at Salaspils] the ground is crying.")

Introduction

Psychoanalytic practices are gradually coming to include the analysis of transgenerational transmission of destructive aggression in their theoretical and technical praxes. This presentation starts off with ordinary and extraordinary stories of *returning to oneself* as part of the narrative on transgenerational transmission. With the return to oneself in mind, I will ask: What basic conceptual assumptions could facilitate how we theorize transgenerational transmission? What *impediments* present themselves when we use existing psychoanalytic theories in inflexible ways as points of entry into psychoanalytic exploration? What may we come to grasp if, for example, we treat some forms of resistance as opportunities rather than opposition to analytic understanding? What, consequently, would constitute analytic readiness to receive the phantoms of transgenerational haunting when they return? These are some of the questions with which we will have to come to grips in order to represent, theorize, and reconfigure the idea of transgenerational haunting so that we may facilitate healing. A transgenerational object relations theory could then be proposed at the end.

The Return of the Subject to Oneself; *or,* *Foreshadowing the Concept of the* Advenant

This chapter will serve as a bridge in two respects: a bridge between theory and practice and, secondarily, a bridge between African American

DOI: 10.4324/9781003389026-6

and Jewish American experiences. The ethical standpoint subserving this bridge is also two-fold. First, although African American and Jewish experiences are not interchangeable, they are horizonal; they tell us what heinous things human beings are capable of doing to each other (see Apprey & Stein, 1998). Second, human beings are defined by their capacity to overturn and to reconfigure the received. The theory of technique for upending the transgenerational transmission of destructive aggression in this book rests on this ethical position. Before entering into that domain, let us feed our imagination with the following three stories.

I

First, it is 1996, five years after the fall of the Soviet Union and the restoration of independence for Estonia. I am in Estonia as part of an interdisciplinary team of American scholars and diplomats who have come ease tensions between Indigenous Estonians and Estonian Russians after Sovietization. There is a break in peace-making proceedings. I decide to take a taxi to visit Salaspils, a notorious extermination camp in Latvia. In the words of Trudy Ulmann Schloss (1991), Camp Salaspils "was *a horrible place* from which *only very few returned*" (p. 60). I have now arrived by taxi at Camp Salaspils. The taxi driver has his orders from a gatekeeper at the death camp and mass cemetery. He may not drive in. I have to walk all alone into the death camp. Unexpectedly, I am seized with terror. I am immobilized. From where I am standing I can see the "cars" in which hundreds were burned to death. From where I stand, an image of *"the door of no return" in Cape Coast Castle comes to me.* Cape Coast castle is a slave castle in Ghana, the country of my birth, from where hundreds of thousands of kidnapped people were bound in chains and ferried in their fetters to the United States. With the condensation of what I am physically seeing and that which I have now conjured up in my head, these words come to mind: *"if anything happened to me here, and if I did not return, no one would ever know."* Upon the translation of my terror into a narrative, I wake up from my temporary simulation of death, and I am able to walk into the death camp alone. When death leaves its traces, none of us can remain unaffected. It was not until I *had returned home* in a phenomenal and experiential way that I could be free to walk and to walk in. When I returned to my physical home in the United States, I looked up the translation of the words that greet visitors at the gate of the death camp at

Salaspils: *AIZ SIEM VARTIEM VAID*. These words translate into English as: *BEYOND THESE GATES THE GROUND IS CRYING*. I had intuitively joined the crying dead when I felt immobilized at the gate.

II

Second, it is the year 2009. A third-year psychiatric resident comes to my office for supervision on a psychotherapy case. He is quite distraught. Why? He has just come out of a clinical seminar where he has finished presenting a first session of a case to his peers and the faculty of child and family psychiatry at the University of Virginia School of Medicine. His medical colleagues ask him to report the case to the local social services for suspicion of child abuse, and he vehemently disagrees with what he considers a premature mandate. What is on the videotape that upsets the faculty and his peers so much? In that first videotaped session, the child opens the shirt of his young psychiatrist and rubs his hands against his chest.

I choose to take a history from the parents. I hear the following. On the father's side, the four-year-old boy's grandfather was so physically violent to the boy's father that grandmother had to take custody of all four children across the street. On the boy's mother's side, the grandfather was so "evil and mean" that he physically attacked most of his six daughters when he was intoxicated. In addition, he sexually violated two of them. When he tried to sexually attack a third, she fought him. He killed her.

For what, then, did the parents from two separate and violent families recruit each other when they met and chose to marry? When the four-year-old boy's parents married, they consciously vowed to raise their child in a non-violent home. They would be gentle with their son when he was born. They were. Upon his birth he had such a severe case of colic that they put him in their marital bed and did not release him until the day they walked into my office four years later. It was at this interview that I discovered that he was *without words*, only babbling like an infant, and that at pre-school he was beginning to be violent; hence the referral. I insisted that they put him to bed in his own room and that he could sleep alone. They insisted he would not. I prepared them. They did as I had asked. He was able to do so. They came to see me the next day with their "stunning" news.

With my supervision, treatment by the psychiatric resident took a little less than a year to restore him to where he should developmentally be. I saw the parents concurrently. Together, we managed to overturn the return of the composite of the violent paternal grandfather and the twice as violent and incestuous maternal grandfather. The child was not being physically or sexually abused. The victims were one generation removed. The perpetrators were two generations removed. He was unconsciously being nurtured to become like his grandparents. *What gives itself* as the story to be understood is a transgenerational story with *the return of the grandparents in the body of a four-year-old boy.*

III

A final story, to which I will return throughout this chapter. A prominent academic physician, a surgeon, refers his 16-year-old daughter to me. She is oppositional in his eyes and in his wife's as well. She has just learned to drive, and although she is a "very good driver," she stays out until late at night driving her drunken friends home. In the eyes of the 16-year-old, she must ensure that her friends are safely returned home. The father, in his turn, is an elderly academic physician with a reputation for saving lives. I decide to see the daughter twice weekly with a view to starting analysis at some future date if it turns out to be needed. I plan to see the parents monthly throughout this treatment. The parents agree to her work in psychotherapy and look forward to her success in treatment. After two months of seeing no immediate change in his daughter, he and his wife decide to ask me to assist them to send their daughter to "a wilderness camp" where she would be subject to a boot camp–type treatment. What is this well-read man asking me to do? He knows what psychoanalysis is. He was analyzed for some seven years during his education in London by one of Anna Freud's colleagues.

In a very poignant session with the parents, he berates me for focusing on the understanding of developmental and behavioral issues and not enough on his request for the child to go to "a wilderness camp" to be "tamed." His anger gradually turns into sadness. With recalcitrant resignation, he utters these words: "I wish I could push her and the car onto the top of some mountain and leave her there." His very loyal wife adds: "and I would tip it over." I follow up with these words: "and she will die." Father adds: "At least there will be two left." I add: "In contrast to your family of origin where everyone but you perished." Mournful tears fall like I have never seen dropping from a man's eyes. His wife wraps her comforting arms around him.

What have the parents given us? A new version of their history. In the original story, the father's discerning parents, anticipating danger, sent him to London to get his medical education. On his way to London, his entire family was seized by the Nazis. They perished in Auschwitz. Not one survived. When he completed his medical education, he married a German woman. They bore three children.

The sedimentations of history were reactivated in my office. The reactivation entered into the transference and the work of mourning and the meaning of his unconscious recruitment of his German wife were understood. They became freer to parent their daughter differently. She was no longer subject to the mandate to ransom her so that the other two siblings would live. Now she is a prominent violinist *back in Germany*, where she works for a major symphony orchestra.

What do these stories have in common? There is a return where the present unconscious coincides with the past unconscious in the fulfillment of an errand where that errand is as much one's own as it is an errand of an Other. Parenthetically, it is not by accident that the French word for "ghost" is "le revenant": that which returns.

VI

I have used three stories where the ordinary and the extraordinary intersect to feed our imagination about returns in transgenerational haunting and transmission. I shall now describe *impediments to theorizing transgenerational haunting* in psychoanalysis. We shall then look at *prospects for unpacking and theorizing the return*. Then we shall turn to an alternative way to read *"resistance"* in order *to enable us to receive that phantom* (Abraham, 1975) *that returns*. Finally, the idea of the *advenant* is filled in to enable us to see what happens in the middle space between analyst and analysand and what a middle-voiced happening is so that we can represent, theorize, and reconfigure the received transgenerational transmission of destructive aggression in psychoanalysis in order to facilitate healing.

Baldly presented, the operational format of this chapter is as follows. In Part 1, something toxic is injected from an ancestral place and bids us to carry out an errand. In Part 2, I suggest that in order to listen to this invisible and inaudible errand, our conventional understanding of resistance must change from a phenomenon that obstructs knowing and meaning making to one that potentially offers us an opportunity to grasps portals of entry into consciousness. In Part 3, representation is depicted as one of the ways in which ancestral or repressed phenomena give themselves, and they give themselves in the public space between self and other in psychoanalysis. In Part 4, we discover that what once looked like a representation of an errand can appear as a concrete presentation if the analyst is able to foster an analytic space for the subject of the analysis to co-create with the analyst the phenomenal return of oneself to oneself in a primary or original "place" of conflict. Here, we revisit Auschwitz to concretely present *a return of the subject to oneself.* This quiet return of oneself to oneself allows us to reframe Freud's instinct theory in Part 5. In Part 6, we have the beginnings of a transgenerational object relations theory.

None of these observations would be fully realized without the radical change in the analytic handling of resistance as obstruction to a new understanding of resistance as a conduit or portal of entry into consciousness.

Part 1: Impediments to Theorizing: Transgenerational Transmission of Destructive Aggression in Individual Psychoanalysis

What is the mode of transmission in transgenerational transmission of destructive aggression? At the outset, something is *injected* from an anterior source; that something is *housed* in a hospitable place for storage for an indeterminate time; that same something is *suspended*; that something that is stored in this time warp carries *a mandate for an errand* to be carried out. Upon the mandate's urgent/voluntary reception, the subject awaits a suitable new object to reawaken the project so that that project *can return to a public space away from a haunt,* as it were. By this time the subject shall have lost sight of who sent whom. *Active and passive have by now become interchangeable. A middle voice speaks, and yet it does so in an invisible and inaudible way* (Apprey, 1993). At the end of this chapter, we add Claude Romano's (2009) contribution on the subject that returns (*advenant*) to our understanding of transgenerational transmission.

What is the nature of this early ego that receives the mandate to die? Now let us bring in Freud. The ego that receives the intrusive mandate is an early and deep ego that is "not a master in its own house" (Freud, 1917). Freud (1917) recognized in his paper "A Difficulty in the Path of Psychoanalysis" that it is a narcissistic blow when the ego recognizes that it is not a master in its own house, as it were, and that the early ego is subject to the dictates of interior and external forces. This idea of the early and deep ego is a necessary starting point for psychoanalytic accounts of transgenerational transmission. It is pivotal because *the early and deep ego cannot process the world "correctly," and for that reason it is at the mercy of conscious and unconscious parental and ancestral infusions.*

What if the theoretical object of psychoanalysis were built on unpacking phenomenological accounts of *givenness* as well as *interpreted constructs*? Here we must be careful not to make a dichotomy between *pure description* (Husserl, 1913/1983) and *interpretation* as in multiple psychoanalytic traditions. *What if disciplined description were to precede interpretation?* More precisely, *what if we were to treat "resistance" in psychoanalysis not solely as an opponent of meaning-making but as an opportunity that gives yet another story?*

For the theoretical basis of this last question, let us turn next to Georges Politzer (1928/1968) and his critique of the structural theory as a starting point. Politzer saw Freud's creation of the structural theory as an impediment and not as an advance beyond the topography of mind of the period 1897 to 1923. In short, *structural theory*, for Politzer, *resorted to realism, abstraction, and formalism* and in so doing *lost the rich psychology* of the *first person singular: "I."*

Part 2: Remembering and Givenness: Revisiting "Resistance" in Psychoanalysis: Georges Politzer's Critique of the Structural Theory

The psychoanalytic concept of transference was initially treated as though it were inseparable from resistance (Freud, 1905, 1912). Now transference is considered the most indispensable tool in psychoanalytic treatment. Similarly, countertransference was initially treated as though it were an obstacle to treatment. Today the transference-countertransference continuum is considered pivotal to psychoanalytic treatment. *Now it is time to extend the same courtesy to "resistance" so that what is traditionally seen as an opponent to progress in treatment can now be considered, with qualification, an event that gives itself in treatment as access to a private narrative.*

We saw, in the wilderness camp story, a father asking an analyst to treat his 16-year-old adolescent child in psychotherapy. We know of his latent desire to take her back to the wilderness rather than make meaning with me in psychoanalytic treatment. We understood that, in that story, the event of that story gave itself or more specifically, *the presentation of that event before me and with me* created an opening to further understanding. We know now that *the opening turned a concrete presentation of a story into a representation of a life-changing event.* This representation opened the door to the meaning-making in treatment he had originally asked for. Typically, such a clinical story can be understood in psychoanalytic terms from at least three standpoints: resistance, in terms of the parents' opposition to the creation of meaning; transference, in terms of their asking me as a clinician to abandon my role and regress into a concrete, syncretic position as an assassin; countertransference, in terms of my helpless appropriation, albeit temporary, of the father's feelings of hopelessness about his daughter's failure to cooperate with him.

It must be emphasized that a clinical story can be understood from multiple conceptual standpoints. At the risk of stating the obvious or debating ideas that have more or less been resolved, let us refresh our clinical minds with some of these conceptualizations for accessing a clinical story. We must do so before we turn to *why it took us so long to treat the concept of resistance as an opening rather than an obstacle.*

In Freud's work, as construed by Politzer, when a subject resists certain thoughts during analysis, these resisted thoughts express themselves in a dream. These resisted thoughts express themselves in a dream because a force impedes their entry into perceptual consciousness. Because this process of resisting thoughts and impeding their entry into perceptual consciousness is already there and beyond the subject's awareness, it cannot be contrived. Freud's conclusion: the existence of the thoughts must be as real as the resistance. Freud's proof: analysis can overcome the resistance and disclose the hitherto impeded thoughts.

Politzer's rendition of Freud's proof is as follows: (1) real thoughts are present, (2) *real thoughts are blocked by resistance*, (3) real thoughts may not be experienced by the subject, (4) real thoughts can have conscious effects, and (5) real thoughts require a real cause or causes. Therefore, an unconscious location for a real cause that generates real effect(s) has to be posited. *To posit that such resisted thoughts preexisted, the analysis resorts to realism. To posit that a general life force accounts for the resistance resorts to formalism.* For Politzer, then, *it takes such presuppositions of realism and formalism to require the positing of the unconscious as a receptacle for inadmissible ideas.*

What is *Politzer's own reinterpretation of Freud's account* of the unpacking of the dynamic unconscious process? Politzer would privilege (1) description and (2) *sticking very closely to the facts presented to the clinician in the room.* When a subject, then, describes a particular difficult situation that presents itself in a dream, the clarification of both sets of descriptive material would unconceal a subject's wishes, sense of threat, feelings, and attitudes toward the difficult situation without having to depart from the level of meaning presented by the naïve data. Politzer's charge: *"To say that a subject has difficulty in admitting incestuous thoughts and to say that he has resisted them is the difference between a 'human' finding based on [human] drama and a psychological description implying realism and formalism"* (p. xxxiv; emphasis added). Freud's failure to stick to description leads Politzer to call Freud's unconscious a place of *"invented descriptions." All we need to avoid positing the unconscious is the human limitation that a human being cannot be omniscient.*

Absent a theory of the unconscious, what would Politzer's description of dream interpretation look like? First, the manifest content of a dream is but a first level of description. Politzer wants us to think of *the manifest level of a dream as only a "scenic montage" and an unconventional presentation that only partially and incompletely expresses the subject's lived attitude. The latent content of the dream is the legitimate second level of description.* Politzer wants us to think of the latent level as that second level of description that can unconceal the meaning of a lived attitude for the subject. *The description at the latent level reveals an adequate description at the level of meaning for "the first-person being."* Consequently, *a subject cannot live more than can be thought. Politzer calls this notion that a subject cannot live more than can be thought "the hidden assumption of articulate thought."* When, however, psychological analysis insists on completing or exhaustively completing the analysis of a given object or phenomenon, representation will have become privileged over being. Let Giorgi, a phenomenological psychological researcher who wrote a

Foreword to the English language translation of Politzer (1994), drive home the latter's viewpoint as follows:

> Being exceeds knowledge. The human subject is not omniscient and not everything that escapes the subject is available to the analyst. The [concept of] unconscious is not necessary, from Politzer's viewpoint, and a [Politzerian descriptively given] concrete science recognizes this sort of limit.
>
> (p. xxxvi)

We can summarize Politzer's link between the manifest and latent content of a dream as follows. *Whereas the manifest content is the unconventional scenic montage, the latent content is the more complete description at the level of meaning; essence without essentializing the meaning. Whereas the manifest content dramatizes a scenario, the latent content thematizes the patient's narrative of wishes or perceived threats.*

It may seem by now that we have lost sight of the original project, that is, reconceptualizing "resistance" in terms of "an opening" (ouverture) rather than closure, obstacle, or hindrance to meaning-making in treatment. On the contrary, we are in the more decidedly secure position to say that *"the wilderness" in our patient's story is a scenic montage, à la* Politzer, *whose unconventional presentation opens the door to the latent meaning of a father's wish to ransom his first-born so that "there would be two left."* No linguistic analysis of the latent meaning is required. We could almost make what Politzer would call *"a simultaneous translation" between the manifest content and the latent content.*

From psychoanalysis, then, we have resistance as a concept. From phenomenology we have the guiding principle of "givenness." Here we see that *what is "given" is the "wilderness" or the wilderness camp.* If we treat what is given, we have *an opening to a rich, powerful, and haunting story. If we treat the request for help to find a wilderness camp to replace psychotherapy and its meaning-making process, we have resistance.* If we collapse the two, givenness and resistance, as both an invitation to see the narrative in front of us, one that is crying out loud to be told, we encounter the *evential, as in Romano, where the evential is* the reconfiguration of the meanings and impact of an historical event. It is this *reconfiguration from event to evential* that promotes growth and even fosters our arrival at a place where some partial resolution of that historical grievance is possible.

Patients have different degrees of readiness for the latent story. It is our ability to ready ourselves to receive that story that takes us from the scenic montage to the meaningful narrative that the patient gives us in the clinical relationship.

In a theoretical way, what constitutes readiness to receive the new and given narrative? What attitudinal position is needed to receive the phantom that returns?

In order to situate ourselves in a position where we are ready to receive the latent and given story, we need to know an ensemble of phenomenological attitudes between description and interpretation. Before then, let us disclose some basic assumptions behind the way stations between description and interpretation. *Presuppositionless* basic assumptions subserve the attitudinal positioning of either a phenomenological investigator or a clinical psychoanalyst who readies oneself to observe a phenomenon's appearing. When one observes in a disciplined way and according to a praxis that is either based on Husserl's epoche or is a derivative of it, there is mutual *encroachment*, mutual *divergence*, and *negotiations* between the subject that observes and the object of the observation. In reverse, the object of the observation causes the subject that observes to become aware of oneself as a subject whose agency is not always master of its house, as it were. A project of determining *intentionality* therefore includes (1) the essential ingredients of one's directedness upon/toward an object, consciousness of the *aspectual shape* and tilt of a phenomenon's appearing, as well as (2) what the observing of the object does to the subject that observes. When one investigates a phenomenon, there is *a necessary tension between pure description and interpretation* as one strives to unpack it in the public space between the observer and the observed.

Equipped with an attitudinal position of *presuppositionlessness*, a readiness to observe how subject and object *encroach* upon each other, *diverge* or *negotiate meaning* in the clinical situation, and most importantly, *what intentionality accompanies the subject's transference wishes*, we can give up Politzer's realist view of Freud's Unconscious with a capital "U" as a concrete and reified place and keep that which is unconscious in perceptual consciousness.

The second adjustment we have to make in Politzer is to modify his rejection of the structural theory by making use of Freud's account of the "ego" in his paper "A Difficulty in the Path of Psychoanalysis" (1917). This ego precedes the ego of 1923–1938 that is more organized and structured as an executive function, among others. This ego of 1917 is, according to Freud, "not a master in its own house" and subject to narcissistic attacks. Easily shattered, it is an early and deep ego that is subject to influences from outside: subject to parental influences. We are not in a position to reject wholesale Freud's structural theory either. If we were to do so, how would we account for the unconscious sense of guilt and other considerations that require us to describe conflict between embedded structures of experience?

Representing and theorizing transgenerational transmission, however, requires us to privilege and elaborate Freud's account of the ego of 1917. Haydee Faimberg (2005), André Green (2004), and Claude Romano (2009) will begin that conversation. All three accounts explicitly or implicitly stand on Freud's early ego, which is more plastic than the ego of the structural theory in later Freud.

Part 3: Representing, Theorizing and Reconfiguring the Concept of Transgenerational Haunting in Order to Facilitate Healing in Psychoanalysis

How do traumatic ancestral legacies shape our lives? *Where are the missing narratives that could potentially make the inaudible cries of turbulence audible and the invisible visible? What is the narrative of reactivation?* In the transference wishes of our patients, what demands, pleas, and/or requests are made to us to render palpable that turbulence that is striving to enter our contemporary scene so that healing can take place? I will turn to André Green, Edmund Husserl, Martin Heidegger, and Claude Romano to frame and reframe our questions and our answers to these questions. I shall reference our "*wilderness*" story along the way to feed our imagination. Finally, I shall rework a theory of transgenerational haunting by radicalizing Freud's concept of *source, pressure, aim, and object of the sexual component instinct.* To that end, let us revisit Husserl.

In Husserl's work (1962, 1989), we see an emphasis on the translation of sedimented or "forgotten" *events of history* to a reactivated *sense of history*. In a previous work (Apprey, 2006), I have extended Husserl's account of *sedimentation* and *reactivation* to a third sphere of the *intentional supplement*, where in psychoanalysis we interrogate not the sedimented events of history, not the reactivation but chiefly the *intentionality behind the transference wishes.* These transference wishes have travelled from (1) the domain of sedimented events to (2) a domain of reactivated and appropriated sense of history and now to an intentional sphere where the analyst may be prodded to, invited to, even bullied to join the analysand to overturn the impact of that psychologically toxic sense of history.

I shall now juxtapose two corollary accounts: Romano's account of events and the world of the subject and André Green's account of representation in the interstices between internal and external fields of reference to how the subject situates oneself in the world. I submit that we would advance our knowledge of the world of representation, in psychoanalysis in general and in Green specifically, if we were able to juxtapose the idea of *the subject that returns to itself* in the process of engagement with events as a corollary discourse.

(A) From French Reception of German Phenomenology to Psychoanalysis With André Green as a Representative Model

It was stated earlier that a theory of transgenerational transmission cannot overlook Freud's (1917) statement that the ego is not a master of its own house. Similarly, Freud's idea has consequences for Green (2004). The first consequence of Freud's idea for Green is that because the early ego cannot initially process the world correctly, there must be negotiation between unrepresentable bodily demands and the psychical representations of those bodily demands.

For André Green, then, inner objects have a double existence: an inner and external world. Between these two worlds, it is *representation* that *brings about communication.* Second, *the representational world makes it possible for the analyst to interpret thought.* Third, the capacity for *thought begins with* a child's *attempt to bring together* the initially *unrepresentable bodily experiences a mother cannot meet* in the external world, on the one hand, *with a child's potentially and psychically representable demands,* on the other. Between the *unrepresentable* bodily demands and the child's psychic *representations of its demands,* there lies *a gap that will never be filled* no matter how good a mother is. *The psyche is therefore a conversation in the gap* within that spatial relationship *between two bodies*: *unrepresentable bodily needs* and the potentially *representable demands of the child.*

Another consequence of the early ego's unreadiness to be its own master is that it must depend on an object outside the body to sustain and support its being because of its *premature condition at birth*. Following Heinz Hartmann (1958), Bolk (1926), and Green (2004) suggests that the result of this premature condition at birth will become the matrix of the mind: a matrix that, in turn, will become constituted by the meeting of the psychical representative by which being is realized into existence. This coming to being comes about through the demands of the body and its association with the demands. The association with the demands depends on "what the mind has kept as *traces of former experiences of satisfaction that bear some similarity to the sought-for situation*" (emphasis in original). This concept is in Freud (1900) as perceptual identity, but Green (2004) will use the idea to launch another, his own idea of *the dynamic restlessness of the subject that seeks a co-existence with the object*. Before then, let us see what he does with Freud's notion of identity of perception.

Green sees the co-option between the tension between the child's bodily needs and their associations as a dynamic one because it modifies psychic representatives of the child's demands and the ideational representatives of the drives through a modification of internal and external world. In my view, *the drives and the associations with the demands of the drives reciprocally change the child's internal fields of reference to the external world, and in reverse the external fields of reference change the input to the interior*.

Clinically, parents who unconsciously wished to speak the drives by taking their daughter back to the wilderness manifestly to be tamed but unconsciously to be sacrificed had cathected the "wilderness" as an external field of reference to their interior turbulence and perennial anguish. Reciprocally, their daughter who had stored her parents' deferred anguish unconsciously created a palpable disturbance in the external world in ways that preserved the restlessness of the inner world; *keeping it very much alive. A reciprocal connection between the parents' reactivation and the daughter's appropriation of the toxic history had to be grappled with and understood before me. A reciprocal correction had to be made through an analytic reconstruction of the hitherto heavily sedimented traumatic history*.

Given, then, the immaturity of the early ego and its dependence on an outside object to maintain and sustain its being, how would Green theorize the relationship of the psyche to the three internal agencies—id, ego, superego—of the mind?

He links them as follows: the *id is the paradise of the mother-baby relationship—flesh to flesh; the relationship of the mother to her mother builds up the ego; and the superego represents the father's role as that which ends the two-in-one relationship between the mother and her baby to which she is bodily linked.*

I would clarify *the mother's relationship to her own mother as a building up of the ego* in the following way: *the mother as auxiliary ego to her child whom she is initially physically linked must simultaneously work through the psychical connection to her own mother.* The representation of that psychical connection informs what she consciously or unconsciously proceeds to do with her child. She does so in identification with her mother. *By linking the mother to her mother, we have begun to introduce the idea of three generations to define a subject. Three generations are therefore needed to define the human subject.*

(B) From the French Reception of German Phenomenology to Continental Philosophy With Claude Romano as Representative Model

Turning now to Romano (2009), let us still bear in mind that our starting point is the early ego and the difficulties it has in processing the world "correctly." In the face of the ego's immaturity, how does the subject translate events into a sense of history (Husserl) or in Romano, how does the subject translate an event into the new configuration that he calls "evential"? In the face of the ego not being a master in its own house, who owns whom and what forms of dispossession are there? In the course of the reconfiguration of the subject's sense of selfhood, what happens to activity and passivity? What structural delay accompanies the reconfiguration?

Event and Evential

He distinguishes between two types of *event*. When *events* happen, they actualize a possibility that is already present in the world, like lightning. On the other hand, events as *evential* overturn existing possibilities and in so doing *reconfigure* the world. In Romano's own words, in the evential reconfiguration, "*the one* who understands is strictly implicated in the very act of understanding: I can understand an event as being addressed to me only if I am myself in play in the possibilities it assigns to me [me destine] and through which it makes history by opening a destiny for me" (p. 30; emphasis in original). There is therefore a system of mutual implications between the event as fact and the one to whom the event happens and for whom, therefore, the evential event, says Romano, is not a fait accompli. It is not inscribed in time and therefore can open up to a movement of futurition. By not being inscribed in time, the subject of the evential can exercise a structural delay, thereby making it accessible from its own posterity from an-archic welling up from nothing, whereas in Green (2004), the timelessness of re-shapes what that event does to him or her or means.

The Unconscious brings up the paternal function to provide order, generalization, and continuity, Romano's *evential* that is not inscribed in time and opens up a movement of futurition that exercises a structural delay that in turn brings about what I will now call "*a pluperfect latency.*"

Romano's phenomenology of the evential suggests that during the reconfiguration of a subject's world, *a metamorphosis that is impossible to date* takes place. Once an event is brought about, it is already too late. We are never contemporaries of its actualization. *We can experience it when it has already taken place*, and this is why, says Romano, an event in its eventness happens only according to *the secret of its latency*. Accordingly, an encounter is not the datable fact of the meeting of two beings but rather that which *lies in reserve* in this meeting and which gives it its future loading. The subject, therefore, is *an advenant* that comes back to oneself. The subject that returns to a prior latency *shall have come back* to oneself after revealing *the secret that lies or has lain in reserve.*

Eventials are not datable. Their secrets lie in reserve. After exercising *a structural delay*, the subject of eventials returns to a prior latency, or more correctly to a pluperfect latency after *the subject shall have come back to oneself* as *advenant*. In this back and forth, past and present, subject and object oscillate in a series of vicissitudes with progressive and retrogressive steps. In Romano's own account, Passibility is "being exposed beyond measure to events that cannot be expressed in terms of passivity but [passibility] *precedes the distinction between active and passive*" (2009, p. 72; emphasis added).

The Evential and the Proneness to Mis-Representation

What, then, makes us so vulnerable to mis-representation? Romano gives us a handle on this with his account of *birth, naming*, and *dispossession of self*. For Romano (2009), to be born is to be connected to history. I am not my own origin. Mine is a destiny all too laid out and pre-assigned to me. So, poignantly, for Romano (2009) "if I cannot take over this past, if this pre-personal past, coming before all memory and forgetting, preceding birth and opening to it, is *a pluperfect I always 'come after'*; it is also what makes possible always 'go before' me and thus well up from the future (p. 78; emphasis added).

To be born, then, is to have a history before having *one's own* history. There is a pre-personal history the subject-as-advenant cannot take over. The subject-as-advenant cannot take over the history of Auschwitz. She would, however, participate with degrees of ownership in a human adventure imbued with excessive meanings that is incommensurable with her projections, projections that are radically inexhaustible. Born into a human adventure imbued with excessive meaning, the subject now has to be named. In what Romano (2009) calls "the inaugural dissymmetry of naming, "*to be named is to be anticipated* by *the verbal initiative of another*, called by a word that overhangs me and that I cannot completely appropriate, *since my name, symbol of my **ownership**,* [symbol] *of my 'identity' is at the same time, symbol of this initial **dispossession**"* (p. 80; emphasis added).

Through *the inaugural dissymmetry of naming*, then, my name is just as much a symbol of my ownership as it is a symbol of my dispossession. We are, however, a little ahead of ourselves here. There is a dispossession of birth that precedes naming as yet another symbol of dispossession. How may we separate these two types of dispossession? Phenomenologically, we may link the dispossession of birth to that which is *"originary"* [sic]. We may link the second dispossession of naming to that which is *"original"*: original because the subject is now capable of self-projecting and capable of participating in a human adventure that is saturated with multiple, excessive, and radically inexhaustible meanings.

Part 4: Back to Auschwitz

The Nazis are preparing to execute Polish Jews. A discerning family saves a son by sending him to London to train to become a physician. He marries a German woman. They raise three children; the oldest of whom must now be *ransomed* so that *two would be left*. Psychotherapy allows the adolescent and her parents to both represent what had hitherto lain *in reserve* until it became *representable* and until we could *reconfigure the sedimentations of history that had been reactivated in treatment and extended to serve a new and contemporary purpose.* A father and mother brought me *a transference wish* that *I could not meet*: a wish to join them *to send their daughter to the wilderness.* This is *simultaneously a transference wish and a phenomenological event.* It is a transference wish to this effect: "please join us as we revisit the wilderness where grandparents perished." It is a phenomenological event to this effect: "The incineration is not datable; its secrets lie in reserve. Once we get past the wilderness story we may be able to represent and reconfigure anew a project that does not kill." An adolescent daughter *could not represent* or reconfigure on her own and by herself what unrepresentable project had been injected into her. Rather, she created an *errand*: a *mistake*, a *wandering, an unconscious errand that had already taken place.* It was her new project to independently and singlehandedly save her endangered friends from death.

In *a pro-ject of **possibility**,* she was an advenant, a sub-ject that had been chosen to be ransomed, as it were, to save the other two siblings, and simultaneously a sub-ject who must rescue others from danger. Thanks to the work of psychotherapy, the return of the daughter to the wilderness was aborted. Now a world-class cellist in her own right, *the **parental pro-ject has been overturned and upended** by the **sub-ject**.* Now she can become a *subject (without a dash) with greater agency* in her selfhood.

Our clinical story tells us that the subject-as-advenant is a vulnerable figure who can be returned to the wilderness, as it were, to be ransomed so that others may live. We are now in a position to say that *fettered to history*, the *advenant is eminently the subject of* utter *misrepresentation.* More accurately, we may say that the subject is both represented and misrepresented, representable and misrepresentable according to the intentionality behind the reactivation and the translation from the events of history to a sense of history.

Part 5: Returning to Freud to Link Freud's Theory of Instinct to the Transgenerational Transmission of Destructive Aggression in Order to Propose a Transgenerational Object Relations Theory

In Freud's *Instincts and Their Vicissitudes* (1915), an instinct has a *source*, it operates under *pressure*, it has active and passive *aims*, and it has an *object*. By the *source* of an instinct, Freud meant a process of excitation that occurs in an organ. This is essentially of a biological and/or chemical nature. By the *pressure of* an instinct, Freud meant the amount of force, peremptory urge, or demand for work, which it represents. By *aim*, Freud meant the direction—passive or active—that effects the bodily change that is felt as fulfillment or satisfaction. The *object* is the thing or figure through which the instinct or instinctual trend achieves its aim. We can now radicalize the world of instincts and instinctual trends into a phenomenological world as follows: The *source of turbulence* is an ancestral world, an anterior (m)other, a prior autochthony that hides a secret desire and renders it latent. The *pressure accompanying the reactivation* need not invariably be urgent or peremptory; rather, it is potentially a slow and insidious one that is passed through the generations. In the process of reactivation, *subject and object oscillate*; subject becomes cast under cover, "thrown under a bus," as it were. Subject gathers itself, binds itself in protest or in recalcitrant resignation, and/or chooses one's own poison if one is perceived to be mandated to die. Finally, the figure of an object through which or through whom the fulfillment is to be derived can *store, suspend, defer*, or *inject* the toxic representation or aberrant mis-representation into yet another sub-ject: a suitable figure that can provide an object home for the mediating subject.

Part 6: Provisional Transgenerational Object Relations Praxis

When we are able to acknowledge the source of the internal turbulence as ancestral when we are able to appreciate the slow and insidious ways in which the phantoms emerge; when we can see that subject and object, passive and active do change places; and lastly, when we can treat the object as a figure that has been recruited to bring us back to ourselves, we would be ready to see both the mysterious and the everyday features of the uncanny. This discovery of the uncanny as both mysterious and ordinary shows itself through *historical events* that are *staged* inside the analysis in the form of *new events* in front of our very eyes and in very palpable ways. Our readiness to treat these events *as givenness to tell an untold story* rather than as opposition to meaning-making brings the subject of an analysis face to face with the phantom.

The analytic subject, then, in this transgenerational praxis, is the one who

1   *embodies the phantom that seeks to return* to a hostile or hospitable place,
2   *gives intentionality to the errand to fulfill a mandate to die or seek ransom,* and
3   *returns to oneself* (*advenant*) in the *new and public space* of the analyst–analysand relationship.

This new space is saturated with *transference wishes, pleas,* or *demands* made by the subject in order to entertain the possibility of *a reconfiguration that fosters healing.*

References

Abraham, N. (1975). Notes on a phantom. In *The Shell and the Kernel*. Chicago: University of Chicago Press, 1994.

Apprey, M. (1993). Dreams of urgent voluntary errands and transgenerational haunting in transsexualism. In *Intersubjectivity, Projective Identification and Otherness*, eds. M. Apprey & H. Stein. Pittsburg, PA: Duquesne University Press.

Apprey, M. (2006). Difference and the awakening of wounds in intercultural analysis. *Psychoanalytic Quarterly*, LXXV: 73–94.

Apprey, M. & Stein, H. F. (1998). Ruptures in time. In *Blacks and Jews on the Couch: Psychoanalytic Reflections on Black-Jewish Conflict*, eds. A. Helmreich & P. Marcus, pp. 102–120. Westport, CT: Praeger.

Bolk, L. (1926). *Das Problem der Menschwerdung*. Jena: Fischer.

Faimberg, H. (2005). *The Telescoping of Generations: Listening to the Narcissistic Links between Generations*. London & New York: Routledge.

Freud, S. (1900). Interpretation of dreams. In *Standard Edition*, Volume 5. London: Hogarth Press.

Freud, S. (1905). Fragment of an analysis of a case of hysteria. In *Standard Edition*, Volume 7. London: Hogarth Press.

Freud, S. (1912). The dynamics of transference. In *Standard Edition*, Volume 12. London: Hogarth Press.

Freud, S. (1915). Instincts and their vicissitudes. In *Standard Edition*, Volume 14. London: Hogarth Press.

Freud, S. (1917). A difficulty in the path of psychoanalysis. In *Standard Edition*, Volume 15. London: Hogarth Press.

Green, A. (2004). *André Green at the Squiggle Foundation*. Edited by Jan Abram. London: Karnac Books.

Hartmann, H. (1958). *The Ego and the Problem of Adaptation*. New York: International Universities Press.

Husserl, E. (1962). *Ideas I: General Introduction to Pure Phenomenology, Book 1*. Translated by W. R. B. Gibson. New York: Collier Books (Orig. 1913).

Husserl, E. (1983). *Ideas Pertaining to a Pure Phenomenology and to a Phenomenological Philosophy, Book 1*. Translated by F. Kersten. The Hague: Martinus Nijhoff (Orig. pub. German 1913).

Husserl, E. (1989). *Ideas Pertaining to a Pure Phenomenology and to a Phenomenological Philosophy, Second Book: Studies in the Phenomenological Constitution*. Translated by R. Rojcewicz & A. Schuwer. Collected Works, Volume 3. Dordrecht: Kluwer Academic Press (Orig. 1952).

Politzer, G. (1968). *Critique des Fondements de la Psychologie*. Paris: Presses Universitaires de France (Orig. pub. French 1928).

Politzer, G. (1994). *Critique of the Foundations of Psychology: The Psychology of Psychoanalysis*. Translated by M. Apprey. Pittsburgh, PA: Duquesne University Press (Orig. 1928).

Romano, C. (2009). *Event and World*. New York: Fordham University Press.

Schloss, T. D. (1991). A farm called Jungfernhof. In *The Unfinished Road: Jewish Survivors of Latvia Look Back*, collected & ed. G. Schneider, pp. 57–59. Westport, CT: Praeger.

Chapter 6

Difference and the Awakening of Wounds in Intercultural Psychoanalysis

In many analyses, patients and analysts alike consciously or unconsciously wound each other. In intercultural analyses, these woundings may take on an extra bite. The author suggests that treatments can be viewed according to the following phenomenology: There are (1) sedimentations of history, which are (2) reactivated and (3) subsequently extended to serve new and contemporary purposes via the inscription of intentionality. If the analysis is well presided over, the violence of difference may reveal significations that exceed the particular, entering into a general and transcendent sphere. Concrete and syncretic matter becomes symbolic and produces a transformation from the primitive origins of a phenomenon to new, motivated, and plural structures of experience.

Introduction

Three basic assumptions subserve the account of intercultural psychoanalysis given in this chapter. First, it is suggested that *human beings reveal their most intimate secrets through the exceptions, but they freeze that which appears to be an exception long enough for us to see ourselves in it*. In this respect, intercultural analysis gives us vivid access to particular human experiences and, in turn, informs other clinical experiences. Second, in the translation from *the events of history* to *a sense of history* (Husserl, 1997), analysands take the sedimentations of history, reactivate them in the transference, and add an intentional dimension that carries the plea, demand, warning, or admonition of which they want their analyst to take notice. Third, in dark and primal caverns of our minds, *difference is simultaneously a provocation and an invitation to push the analyst to remember with the analysand*. In this respect, taking the negative transference, housing it, and transforming it is a privileged technical aspect of intercultural psychoanalysis.

DOI: 10.4324/9781003389026-7

Before venturing further into the field, let us hear three voices from two patients and a psychoanalytic candidate in order to fire our imaginations.

1   "I am scared of you. You are an African. You will eat me up."
2   "You are like the native aborigine—in the movie *Walkabout*—who rescues a boy and his sister after their parents kill each other. He taught them how to survive in the wilderness."
3   "Where do you get off speaking knowledgeably about the Holocaust? You are very polished. You have not suffered."

Michel de Certeau (1997), the French human science scholar and author of *Heterologies: Discourse on the Other*, considered that what is foreign is that which escapes from a place. In the first quotation previously, the foreigner who escapes is a presentation, not a representation, of *the cannibal*. In the second, a representation escapes: a foreigner who rescues after the presentation of a double murder. In the third, sadistic envy escapes, driven forcibly into a foreigner who dared to give speech to an unspeakable crime: the slaughter of millions of human beings.

Here are de Certeau's (1997) elaborative comments:

> *What is foreign is* first of all the "thing." It is *never where the word is.* The *cannibal* is only a variant of this general difference, but a typical one since he is *supposed to demarcate a boundary line.* Therefore, when he sidesteps the identifications given him, *he causes a disturbance that places the entire symbolic order in question.* . . . The cannibal is the figure on the fringe who leaves the premises, and in doing so jolts the entire typographical order of language.
>
> (pp. 70–71, italics added)

We might note that my two patients and the analytic candidate quoted previously "signify not the reality of which they speak, but the reality from which they depart" (p. 71).

Why am I discussing this? In the world of intercultural analysis, *difference may not be tolerated.* Black and white quintessentially are opposed. In this world, there are evocations of *lacerations, injury, wounds, murder, assassinations.* This is a *concrete, material world, a dark place* where, to paraphrase the poet Georges Blin's adage (1945), that which has integrity constitutes a provocation to us (p. 44). Gaston Bachelard (1943) would add that "One might debate endlessly the primacy of sadistic instinct or seductive images in this response. One might say, in support of the first view, that sadism actively seeks out objects to carve up, to wound" (p. 28). In such a world, then, instincts awaken in us an incisive will—a will to cut, to wound the other. Bachelard would add (wisely yet again): "This kind of sadism acts under cover, beyond the reach of the *superego*" (p. 28, italics in original).

Now that I have sufficiently triggered the reader's imagination about the richness of intercultural psychoanalysis, allow me to explore this theme systematically with you.

Evoking Husserl and Bachelard

Let us turn to the first patient quoted previously, a British psychotic anorexic who feared that her African clinician would eat her up. We could say that her own cannibalistic greed had gotten the better of her precisely *because* she was anorexic. This way of viewing experience as driven by the causal context of nature compelled Husserl (1997) to coin the term *naive psychologism*. In this respect, as a native of Ghana, I am a cannibal because an anorexic who breaks down into psychosis can construct an African only as a black cannibal, one whose meaning is constructed by her using the imagery of darkness, the unknown, into which she can ascribe a sinister intentionality. We live in the same world, but she has chosen to intentionally situate herself as one who can be voraciously taken into an other's body as victuals, digestible food, which in turn could awaken murderous phantoms that dwell inside her. Her life is in peril. She has closed off all possibilities that I could be helpful to her, a good guest inside her body, as it were.

Suppose, then, that we try to transcend this naive psychologism, that mode of experiencing that is grounded in the causal and biological context of nature. Suppose that we view our white psychotic's way of situating herself in front of a dark-skinned clinician as based on previous sedimentations of darkness perceived as unknown and dangerous. These sedimentations are *transcendental* for Husserl (1997) because they are distributed over all aspects of our life-world: economic ("it was a dark day on Wall Street today"), historical, political, social, and so on. Here there are oscillations between passive and active generation. There is a doubling of associative links, so that anything actively created and subjectively constituted by my patient depends on previous sedimentations of life experiences that now lay passively dormant in her consciousness and mine. Such sedimentations of prior acts of construction have traditionally been considered unsuitable for psychological inquiry; rather, they have been seen as belonging to the realm of philosophy.

There is another possibility to consider if we wish to conduct a psychological investigation of how our patient views blackness, eating voraciously, and so on. We may consider that: (1) there are *sedimentations* of history, (2) these sedimentations are *reactivated* in the transference in ways that suggest an oscillation between active and passive generation, and (3) *intentionality* is inscribed as a part of that reactivation.

Thus, we have a three-tier ascension from sedimentation to reactivation to intentionality. We are now in the realm of psychoanalysis. In this clinical sphere, the following points hold true:

- for every *event* of history, there is a *sense* of history;
- for every physical materiality, there is a functional correlate;
- for every physical presentation, there is a psychical representation.

Therefore, we must seek commonalities between antinomies of:

- inside–outside
- essences–accidents
- reality–appearance
- center–structure
- natural–cultural
- centrifugal–centripetal
- intrinsic nature–ostensible nature
- meaning–significance
- mind–world

Bachelard (1939) offers further food for thought:

Literary symbolism and the symbolism that is Freud's, such as they are executed in classical symbolism and normal dreamwork, are only mutilated examples of the symbolizing powers active in nature. Both present an expression that has been arrested too soon. They remain substitutes for a substance or person that deserts evolution, *syntheses named too quickly, desires uttered too soon.* A new poetry and *a new psychology* that might describe the soul as it is being formed, language in bloom, *must give up definite symbols or images learned merely and return to vital impulses and primitive poetry.*

(p. 31, italics added)

In this respect, then, the concrete/syncretic and the symbolic are continuous. The syncretic can ascend into the domain of the symbolic, and, likewise, the symbolic can descend into the syncretic. What does it mean for me, then, that I am an analyst with a dark skin? The phenomenological element that I carry into intercultural analysis is that, in presiding over an intrapsychic story, I may have a huge advantage as a dark person over others who have to search for the transference. I do not have to look very far for what transference I am being invited to take on when I appear in a patient's dream as an untrustworthy Japanese restaurant owner who uses his restaurant to make families come together. And the transference is ever so transparent when I am an unexpectedly kind, Nigerian army general or when Mount Kenya is erupting with volcanic fire in a patient's dream after an acrimonious session. In the dark, one cannot see. One may be harmed. When my patients enter these dark, epistemic places, their safety is perceived to be at stake, and an ever-so-fortuitous negative transference is evoked. In such primal places, anything that has integrity is a provocation and must be dismantled by the dreamer. I must be ready to absorb, house, and transform the project behind the negative transference in order to advance the analysis.

Such a story follows in this clinical vignette.

A Clinical Story

A French physician comes to see me for psychoanalysis for her suicidal impulses. In the past, she prematurely terminated a Lacanian analysis and two Freudian analyses on both sides of the Atlantic. With a determined disposition, she warns me that I may be the next analyst she fires. With scorn, she discovers that I come from Ghana, West Africa. With cynicism, she tells me her suspicion that I may be like those French analysts who are "all words." She had already Googled me to learn that I had written about French and German phenomenologists, notably Merleau-Ponty and Husserl.

The differences between us are palpable. She is light-skinned; I am very dark-skinned. She has seen the violence of poverty; economically, I have been relatively fortunate. She practically reeks with pain; I carry with me a naive, pre-ambivalent mythology that the world is a basically good place. She is full of hate; I dream of fresh starts in the face of adversity.

Analysis begins with the patient's statement that "I don't want to be here and I want to speak in French."

Sedimentation

The patient talks about "a huge sadness around a big thing." She wants to *eject* her uncooperative young adult children out of her life; she would like them to disappear. She feels like she is in a prison, and she feels empty. In her mind, she tells me, there is a place like a cave to which she retreats when she is in distress. That cave feels like a home.

I will let her speak for herself:

> It's comfortable, I feel safe there, and it's fuzzy. It's like a *uterus* and I can see outside. It tilts deep into the diaphragm. It takes a lot of work to see outside and be inside. *It's at the back; there is a tension between staying inside and outside.* I feel the *tension at the root of the diaphragm.* Then I have this other vision. It's a quick vision of a monster—*a tortured vision of a monster trying to push things out of this cave.*

There is a related dream:

> I was in a maniac [sic] mood, visiting the past—people and places in the past. I was in a cellar. I told myself: "I am glad I am not paying the bills for this cellar because the water is not draining out." There was a floor in the cellar: It was pre-cement, reverse pillars [sic]. In the place where you could have put a pillar, the pillar was not there, and the draining was not happening. So I poked a stick in there. An old structure was blocking the pathway of this water. (She laughs out loud.) And I do remember, I wasn't paying the bill for this place! And I met this woman that I used to know in Belgium. When I hugged her, I felt her spine. She said, "Ugh!" She was so skinny; I could even palpate the front of the vertebrae. *It was deep in the diaphragm.* I could feel

the elasticity, but it wasn't flexible enough. I decided to separate the two vertebrae. "Bloh!"—and it was fixed!

In her associations, the patient wonders if the space between the anus and the vagina, the space that tilts deep into the diaphragm, is the cloaca, and decides it is so. The cloaca is the premammalian organ for excreting digestive, reproductive, and urethral waste matter, she notes. Then she speaks about an old castle that has a round cave with the shape of two eggs touching each other. "Oh, I forgot something majorly [sic]!" she interjects. "When I was going down into the cellar in the dream, there was a bunch of people. There was a young woman like my daughter; and an old woman— a dangerous witch—was there."

I summarize this material to the patient as follows:

> You have a world. It has inhabitants: a maternal figure—call her a witch—who withholds food; a starved person, whose body structure must be fixed; and a daughter who must beware. And you are the person who fixes the starved woman.

The patient elaborates with an old dream that dates back to when her daughter was a baby:

> There was a huge river with a strong current. My daughter had fallen into the water. She was fighting to survive. And so I was telling her, "You can do it! You can do it!" A big woman, a feminine version of Darth Vader—she had a face but not a mask, said: "No, you are not going to do what your mother said. There is a right way to do it [i.e., to come out of water with strong currents]." It was a breakthrough when I realized that all three people were me. The big authoritative woman had become a witch. That doesn't scare me anymore.

This, then, is a sedimented structure of the patient's experience:

1 There is a place to return to when one is in distress.
2 This place, a cave, is safe, comfortable, and fuzzy.
3 However, it feels like prison.
4 In such a habitus, no feeding takes place; the inhabitants are emaciated, even anorexic.

5   The inhabitants must beware.
6   The witch matriarch owns the cellar.
7   She establishes the way one swims against stormy currents.
8   Since the pillars are out of their places and imperfect structures block the draining of water, she, the witch, must pay the bill.
9   The witch owns the body that houses the contents of this habitus.
10 The cloaca—the place of discharge for the intestinal, reproductive, and urinary functions—is not a place where feeding takes place; hence, it has an emaciated inhabitant.

Reactivation

Not long afterward, I learned that the patient worked tirelessly at riding and training 12 horses every day. At the end of one very difficult session with her, as I noticed a very bad taste in my mouth, the longer epigraph of T. S. Eliot's poem "The Waste Land" (1922) suddenly came to me. It speaks of the mythic figure of Sybil sitting in a vessel, reading her rune, in plain sight, and when the boys asked her what she wanted, she answered that she wished to die. In fact, no interpretation could mitigate the patient's self-erasure, until an event that occurred later on: a horse fell on top of her, and "I almost died," in her words. She had broken her pelvis, causing her to miss two weeks of analysis. Upon her return, she said that the following words of mine had "sustained" her: "You must not allow yourself to be ambushed."

The patient gradually worked her way in subsequent dreamwork out of the cave. At the end of the first year, she brought me a gift: *the seeds of a castor oil plant*. Noticing the next day that her gift was still on my desk and still the subject of analysis, she said, rather casually:

By the way, if you decide to take the plant seed home, be careful where you plant it. I don't know if there are children in your house. You must not touch the seeds. It can be a poisonous plant, even though it can grow richly.

In short, it could kill me, my children, or their children if any one of us were to touch the seed.

Now an irresistible quotation from Virgil comes to mind: "Timeo Danaos et dona ferentes." As many will know, it translates as: "I fear the Greeks even when they bring gifts." Our suicidal patient had thus turned assassin. Someone must die. If it were not to be her, it must be me and/or my offspring.

At the beginning of the second year of treatment, we could hear the patient's imagined transformations: Nazi executioners must give up their dark fabrics in favor of Majorcan and colorful African fabrics. She was interested in building models and doing craft work. Structures that she built must have light entering into the interior.

These transformations continued until we hit another difficult patch in our work together, one that lasted nine months. She would set up situations that would cause her to be out of analysis for long periods, and then return and berate me for not being available enough. Or, she would be late by as much as 25 minutes, and then come in to tell me that she had driven 90 miles an hour to get there: "I felt feisty behind the wheel" (said while lying on the couch, throwing her four limbs outward as though she wanted to break out of an enclosed space). Her biggest grievance was that I was either arrogant or uncertain of myself, and so I should seek the help of a clinical supervisor: "After all, all analysts need to have supervisors."

Intentionality

I have discussed sedimentations of historical events (or grievances), as well as reactivation of that which is sedimented. Now a third tier is needed to show that what is reactivated has intentionality: That is, into this third tier is inscribed the motivated behavior—the intentionality—behind what has been reactivated in the transference, in order to serve new and contemporary purposes.

Let us turn now to two sessions at the very beginning of the third year of this patient's analysis.

Pivotal Session I

SHE: I feel like breaking away from you.

I: In the same precarious way that you broke away from your previous analysts?

SHE: I thought about that! (There is a pause, and then she speaks somberly, in the grammar of a child.) I go away because I am scared. *I am scared of being crushed by you.*

I: Scared of being crushed by the figure of an incompetent mother/analyst who cannot keep dates straight and be there for you?

SHE: No-o-o-o, I don't think it's that. I just think there is something in your tone of voice that tells me you are not very happy with my lateness. You know, I never thought about this; my father was like that.

He was always rushing around; always in a rush. But it's not about time so much. In his case, it's about squeezing, not having a place to live.

I: Please continue.

SHE: When he was twenty-five or so, my father was practically squeezed out of his place by his parents. He decided to move out of his father's home because it was untenable for his mother. (pause)

I: (I feel uneasy and unsettled about the disconnected tie between us. I want to explore it, emphasizing the affective side of the relationship.) You are afraid of my crushing you. In addition, someone is being squeezed out of place, and you feel the pressure to break away from me. In an uncanny sort of way, your language tells me that you want to abort the analysis and feel under pressure to do so.

SHE: Maybe my dream will tell us something.

Here is the patient's dream:

> I was in a car, an old Volvo. I was between two vineyards. The car was going, but not with a whole lot of power. There was a mudslide. The mud was falling on the car like an ocean. I woke up in a panic.

And here are her associations to the dream:

> Spencer's son, my stepson, also called Spencer, made a movie about rape. I sent him back a message saying I had been *écoeurée* by his film. I didn't have to use that word. It means "disgusted," but I wanted also to say that my heart had been pulled out. I was *jabbing*. I didn't need to do this.

I: Perhaps. At another level, could you have been *remembering* something?

SHE: I know, I know. An *acte de manqué*, at some level.

I: You responded to the movie as if you had been raped by having to watch it.

SHE: Yes, but now I remember. He had signed the movie *Spencer X*, like it was for his father. The first movie he made was for his mother.

I: Would you feel able to tell me what you saw in the movie?

SHE: It was very disgusting. It took place in an underground garage. A woman is getting inside her car. And at first a man innocuously comes to ask her something. The menace builds up, and then he rapes her. The worst part of it was that she tried to defend herself, and she could not! It gave me this feeling of impotence just to see this disgustingly ugly man rape her.

I: Earlier in this session, a person is scared of being crushed by another: you—by me. Someone is squeezed out of his home: your father. A person is scared. A person is disgusted and her heart is being pulled out; she is jabbing. And rape, an aggressive sexual act, takes place. Now we hear about a mudslide that threatens to kill the occupants of a Volvo. What do you know about the circumstances of your birth?

SHE: I know that I was born with the umbilical cord wrapped around my neck three times. *I know that it was emotionally a big challenge.* I was born on November 19; it is harvest time. You sow also. I was the first to be born of my parents' marriage, and my paternal grandmother thought it was ridiculous to be born in hospital. Those days, in the early '50s, it took one and a half hours to get there. And after all that ordeal, they left my mother there alone in hospital. My grandmother didn't stay. On Sundays, she came to visit. *They* left my mother because they said they had work to do. (The patient cries profusely.) The midwife consoled my mother. So that's what I know about my birth. I was born by forceps.

I: Kicking your way out of the vulva in a mudslide, in an "ocean" of blood. Kicking and jabbing to be let out as your mother tried to squeeze you out of the birth canal, trying to free yourself from the cord that tied you to your mother.

SHE: Oh, yeah—I was blue.

I: This African midwife, so to speak, has news for you: you have already survived, even though, from time to time, I see you kicking and making fists on the couch when you are feeling feisty about something.

SHE: Good, yeah, good. I survived, and I did better with my children. Except my son had the cord around his neck, too. And there's a part of him that is not alive. (pause) You are away in November and I am away for six weeks after you come back. (Fretting over my having gone away some nine months ago, she asks me if I would let her know all the times in the coming year that I will be away. I let her know then that I will be away for an extensive time: three weeks in November. A month earlier, she informed me that she could not arrange a series of family meetings overseas to coincide with my time away.) *I don't know what I am going to do without you.* (She pauses. There will be time to analyze this willful resistance on her part, but this is not the time; this is a time for accurate empathy, genuineness, and even non-possessive warmth—not the time for an interpretation that might be perceived as punitive. She speaks again, chuckling.) The *Volvo* sounds like the *vulva*, doesn't it?

I: And the pathway between the two vineyards is like the birth canal, with an ocean of blood/mudslides blocking your way out of it.

SHE: That pathway between the two vineyards was a very familiar sight of my growing up. I did a lot of work in these spaces that are sort of wasted, because—if you think of it just from the economic point of view—you make a road, and you have room only for a tractor to come through. (pause) Thank you for your *bienveillance* (that is, for my being awake while she slept).

I: It is also for me to thank *you*, for trusting me with the story of your birth.

Discussion

There is a great deal to be understood here. The patient wants me to get a supervisor to oversee her analysis. Her mother was left alone, "unsuper-vised," as she tried to give birth to her daughter. The patient wanted me to be supervised as she prepared to tell me the story of her birth, so that I could preside over the rebirth more competently. And in reactivating the sedimentations of history, she went one step further: "Do not leave me like my grandmother did."

This patient set out to force me to abort her analysis. She provoked me in every way she knew—and she knew it. She would come in very late after speeding on the highway, having risked her life and others', claiming she enjoyed the "feistiness" involved in careening past other drivers. As she provoked me, I stood still. At times, I felt very competent to deliver her. At other times, I felt I was not doing my best work; now I can surmise what my uneasiness was about.

I was like a mother who in the patient's eyes was incompetent to deliver her. What would this "delivery" mean: A physical delivery from her mother? A psychical delivery? When I said to her that I had news for her, to the effect that she had already been safely delivered, it was a way of letting her know ahead of time that this was not the end of the story. *The fight to break out of the vaginal canal served the purpose of survival. Now that fight had taken on a secondary autonomy, so that she was fighting to live even when there was no need to fight.* As a result, I expected her to fight me now and then, again and again, until she found new and creative adaptations that bespoke her psychological birth, permitting her to develop with greater integration. Witness her phrase: "I feel split most of the time. I am one person here. The light is on one part of me; one part cannot be with the other."

Pivotal Session 2

Just before the next session I will describe, I was at a meeting in London for two weekdays and a weekend. Upon my return, I had canceled another two weekdays in order to be in New York for a case presentation. All together, I had canceled four of the patient's sessions. She had erroneously come to her first canceled session on the previous Thursday.

SHE: I came on a day that I should not have come. I knew you were not here. *No*—I had forgotten you were not here. I was really anxious. I felt guilty. Maybe I did something.

I: As if it were your fault that the umbilical cord was wrapped around your neck three times—feeling guilty, as if you had decided how you were to be born.

SHE: (grunts) Ugh. I see that in my daughter Sandra. She has the same thing. A little shit happens and she feels guilty.

I: You had been trying to tell me the story of your birth: your mother's difficult experience in giving birth to you for some time. Trying to make me feel as uncertain as she felt. It took time to tell the full story, but you did it.

SHE: (defensively, as if I had attacked her) But I take a lot of time to do things.

I: Progress now becomes learning how you can be generative without wrapping a cord around your own neck, *by your own hand.*

SHE: Well, I have to tell you something. In the dream where I was in this mud . . .

I: Coming at you like an ocean?

SHE: Yeah, your interpretation was absolutely perfect. It was the first time that I felt I didn't have to oppose or resist an interpretation. As much as you feel I doubted your capacity, you must know that I felt that way, that you were on the mark.

I: I passed the test that three previous analysts failed, causing you to fire them.

SHE: (She is very amused. She is energized.) No-o-o. Not three. Four! I told the last one that he looked like Hitler. I was terrible to him because he was Jewish. So now let's talk about the difference between you and them. With the French guy, it was all words. Another one accused me of barging into someone's session when I had been waiting for thirty minutes for him. The Jewish guy who looked like Hitler, I already told you about; and with Dr. X, nothing happened, so I left.

I: I am all ears. Please continue.

SHE: Two things are on my mind now. I had the thought that *Narcissus* . . . I know the concept. . . . I know the story but I can never remember his name without asking you for it. It came to me for the first time without asking for your help to remember his name. *Each time I try to remember this guy's name, I am gasping for air*. I know that that is what I have been grappling with for weeks! I don't think there is a more central issue than this one: my narcissism. Now that makes me anxious that we won't meet for November, December, and part of January.

I: I understand your fear as follows: that while I am away, you could die. Nine months ago, you asked me to tell you when I was going to be away during the whole year. I gave you the information because you wanted to be sure we were both away at the same time on most occasions. And then you proceeded to set things up so that the analysis as a place of psychological birth would be attacked. Nine months ago.

SHE: Really!! (Her voice is excited.)

I: Yes.

SHE: That is uncanny. (long pause) I look forward to seeing my parents in Belgium in December. (long pause) *When I start to talk about Narcissus, it's a topic where I feel at the edge*. You are the analyst. *You as the mother giving birth to a new person*. Would it be possible? I don't know how to do it.

I: When you talk about Narcissus, it is your way of saying that you were at the edge of life and death with an incompetent mother: me as the figure who represents your mother in labor, and me as the person, the analyst, who needs supervision.

SHE: (fiercely) I still think that all analysts should have supervision, but I see your point.

I: Allow me to stay at the level of the unconscious so that we can together grasp what you have been telling me these past nine months: you needed me to act incompetently; you pushed me hard to not feel like an expert, to have the feeling of being an imposter that a young mother has. But, with the help of your dreams and the analysis, we managed to avoid a stillbirth.

SHE: I know now. I almost did it again. I almost wrecked another analysis. But I don't think I would have. I am tired.

I: You can rest. I will be here.

SHE: In a way, I feel like a speck of something. I feel like I am now a huge, furry animal. (laughs out loud) One day, I had a dream. I had it when I came to Colorado, back in 1979. And this dream has stayed with me very, very vividly: a furry animal crossed my path. I was walking in a forest. The forest was moving with its body and with the air. I felt like it was *a sense of* my mother and also *the reality of the forest*. It was very, very real.

I: It had an impact on you.

SHE: I don't even know why I am telling you. I felt like I was in pieces, in an unclear way.

I: Perhaps it felt like the way a newborn child might feel. Psychologically, you are not sure whether you are whole or in pieces, a whole child or a furry animal, boy or girl, dead or alive, asleep or awake, carried in the air by your mother or of your own free will.

SHE: Yeah! Yeah! (pause) I want to start painting again. Yesterday I went to a room that I want to renovate for my painting. I felt shitty. But I spent three hours listening to Yo-Yo Ma. I love the cello. And it was really good. It felt good to be in that space, to be alone in there. I did a collage just to have a sense of the work I'd be doing there. It was a great complement to the work I am doing here. (pause) You know my thing of *cleaning out*, cleaning out everything? I did a barn sale. It was the farm manager's idea. We work well now; I work with him quite well now. We had a sale on Saturday. We had a lot of fun. We didn't sell much.

I: But I hear satisfaction in your voice that *the cleaning out was good.*

SHE: And the funny thing was that, on Sunday, my husband came to say, "I want you to keep this and that." It was just like him—deciding to get rid of something and then asking to keep it.

Conclusion

The concrete is a necessary starting point. It is a potential starting point for a clinical story, one that necessarily takes the *events of history* and transforms them into a *sense of history*. In such an appropriation of history, the cloacal function is a concrete expression of getting rid of waste matter from the digestive, reproductive, and urinary tracts in the premammalian world. In the sedimentations of this patient's historical grievances, she is able to invoke cloacal imagery to clean out her wounds, as a starting point. When these sedimentations enter into the transference, one of us must be ejected. One of us must die, but somehow we both survive. As a result, I am invited to become a delegate for an incompetent mother, who in turn must be supervised to carry out her psychological birth.

The three-tiered notion of sedimentation, reactivation, and the intentional dimension provides us with a heuristic model for presiding over an intrapsychic story in psychoanalysis, interracial or otherwise. The transference and its use of concrete/syncretic imagery is but one distinguishing element in interracial analyses. The dark is a real place in the world in which we all live. It shows up at night. It also has a personal meaning for each of us. Under regression, we enter into a place where *that which is different and has integrity is a provocation.* Predator anxiety can be evoked. It can take on an extra bite: a metaphor for some of us, an extrojection of cannibalistic impulses for our regressed patients.

What was the exit strategy for my patient from the "dark and *syncretic* presentation?" She painted her answer in a *symbolic* representation for me. Three years after the analysis, she brought me a painting. It was a painting of a man at the helm of a canoe. A lady sat in the middle of the *transport*. "This is how I saw our work together: *You helped me cross a river*." This time, her gift, unlike the castor oil plant she brought me after one year of analysis, and which I only interpreted at that time within the intrapsychic story of the analysis, was now symbolized. This time, I thanked her and I accepted the material gift *in se* and the symbolized gift of our *collaboration*.

References

Bachelard, G. (1939). *Lautreamont*. Dallas, TX: Dallas Inst. of Humanities Publications, 1979.

Bachelard, G. (1943). *Earth and Reveries of Will: An Essay on the Imagination of Matter*. Dallas, TX: Dallas Inst. of Humanities Publications, 2002.

Blin, G. (1945). L'entaille. *Poesies*, 28(October–November): 44.

de Certeau, M. (1997). *Heterologies: Discourse on the Other*. Minneapolis, MN: University of Minnesota Press.

Eliot, T. S. (1922). *The Waste Land and Other Poems*. New York: A Harvest HBJ Book.

Husserl, E. (1997). The Amsterdam lectures. *Husserliana*, 9: 301–348.

Chapter 7

Reinventing the Self in the Face of Received Transgenerational Hatred in the African American Community

There are many clinical methods for understanding and transforming the impact of historical trauma and reinventing the self in the clinical process. However, the approach advocated here requires that regardless of what clinical method of intervention is chosen, a particular strand must run through the process of treatment to produce durable and meaningful change. This strand must run through psychoanalysis, creative and expressive arts therapies, as well as many forms of intervention in aggrieved communities. The strand includes understanding human suffering, the way that particular suffering is mentalized by the victimized group and subsequently reenacted by generations to come. In technical terms there must first be many profiles of understanding of the historical injury. Then there must be an understanding of how the aggrieved community has stored in their communal memory those psychological hurts—those feelings of humiliation and changing historical accounts of the actual injuries. Subsequently those sedimentations of historical grievances are enacted within the transference in the clinical situation where the grievances are not only staged, but re-staged, distorted, or extended. Then comes the most decisive obligation the clinician has towards the analysand, patient, client, or community that is attempting to transform itself. That decisive obligation is to extract the errand or ambush towards extinction and to undergo the unpleasant drudgery of constantly engaging the mandate to die or destroy oneself in order to find new and more flexible forms of adaptation.

Introduction

The French phenomenologist and social science scholar Jean Francois Lyotard (1991) has suggested that in order to understand history, we might

DOI: 10.4324/9781003389026-8

wish to escape the impasse of necessity and total freedom, the rationality of history, and the contingency of it. In other words, to the extent that history can be unique, necessary or inevitable, it can have "a meaning" (p. 131). History also has "some meaning" (p. 131) that may be collective. In this sense Lyotard (1991) writes:

> This collective meaning is the result of the meanings projected by historical subjectivities at the heart of their coexistence, and which these subjectivities must recover in an act of appropriation that puts an end to the alienation or objectification of this meaning and history, constituting in itself a modification of this meaning and proclaiming a transformation of history.
>
> (p. 131)

For this reason, Lyotard suggests that there is not objectivity or subjectivity on one side or the other. There is no objectivity that is heterogeneous, no subjectivity that is all-encompassing. For Lyotard (1991), then, "there is never a total understanding of history" (p. 131), because any historical understanding that is adequate is nevertheless incomplete. Agreeing with Lyotard, I would add that understanding of history that is ethical and engages history in a way that provides a new profile of knowing creates a new future. In order to grasp how transgenerational trauma poisons nostalgia (nostos, GK, return home and algos, pain) we must articulate how the historical pain associated with the exilic condition is mentalized and appropriated so that any sense of homecoming or at-home-ness is destroyed or compromised. I shall propose that the consequences of historical injury lend themselves to particular structures of behavior, some of which poison nostalgia. I shall propose further that the appropriation of the cruelty or the ambush to destroy oneself is intimately tied to the inability to experience genuine nostalgia and therefore to the capacity to deal with the pain associated with nostalgic feelings.

A. Some Basic Assumptions Behind Mentalization of the Impulse Towards Extinction

Tzvetan Todorov, the Hungarian-born human science scholar and director of research at the Centre National de la Recherche in Paris, wrote in

1993 as follows: "Human beings are at once alike and different. . . . The essential thing is to determine just how far the realm of identity extends and where the realm of difference begins; we must try to discover just what relations obtain between the two realms" [that is, of difference and identity] (p. 90). Three years later he became more pointed in his remarks. He said: "If we look at definitions of the human in the mainstream of European thought, we are led to a curious conclusion: the social dimension, the fact that living with others is not generally conceived as being necessary" (Todorov, 1993, p. 1). He wants us to know, however, that this unspoken asocial vision is not the only one but a dominant one.

In my own work (Apprey, 1996a) on interracial conflicts and the need for African Americans to work towards overturning the impact of the consequences of transgenerational transfer of destructive aggression, I have, following Hillis Miller (1992), suggested a four-step heuristic strategy to observe and ultimately transform the received hatred. The following key rubrics will introduce us to the heuristic strategy: (1) line, (2) character, (3) transgenerational haunting, (4) figure.

Under the first rubric of line, we may think of a broken line, a cut, a gap, rupture, lost ancestry, and the wound of an absence in the African American lineage. What attempts, successful or otherwise, are made to suture the wound of an absence? The use of exotic first names juxtaposed to simple European last names like Jones, Williams, or Smith is one example of the attempt to fill the gap. However, we must be careful when we examine the strengths of such creativity intended to fill a gap. Some names unconsciously recreate the very trauma from which a family may be attempting to extricate themselves. A case in point: George Roger Smith is 11 years old. He comes to a treatment center for children for the treatment of his conduct disorder. In the history-taking process, a psychologist, whose prior work I had supervised, chooses to ask how the boy received the names George and Roger. She learns that the child's mother linked the name George to "the mischievous Chicken George" in the movie *Roots* and Roger to 007, who "can get out of all kinds of traps." Prior to answering the question about the naming of her child, the mother had described a mischievous child whom the mother needed to keep indoors for fear that he would leave the house and bring back stolen shoes. When she locks the door, however, he sneaks out of the window and brings up yet one more pair of new sneakers.

Under the rubric of character (Kharassein, GK, to brand) we may think of a scratch, the verbs to engrave, to make a deep impression, to carve, in short, to put a hot rod in a blazing fire—make a deep branding impression on the skin of a slave and, in so branding him, declare the signification "I own you." Or, a Nazi soldier may pin a star of David on the chest of a Jewish person and declare the constructed signification "You are vermin. You must burn." Witness the reversal of agency of branding in the African American community, the extreme case being the extensively tattooed Dennis Rodman with varieties of hair color. Witness the causation of injury and death in black-on-black crime where the African American transgressor has lost sight of the original enemy.

Under the rubric of transgenerational haunting, we come to the transfer of destructive aggression from one generation to the next. In such a transfer we may witness a shift from suicide in one generation, murder in the next, followed by, let us say, incest or physical abuse in a subsequent generation, and so on and so forth. It is as if the injured group has accepted the message that they do not deserve to live and therefore must die in one form or another. At the very least, that injured group may exist in a reduced form such as living but living a most unproductive life. Here the motor of ambush toward one's death remains the same, but the license plate, that is, the form of reducing oneself to nothingness, changes from one generation to the next.

Last, the figure of bartering or exchanging goods that was once perverted into reducing humans to goods must be restored. In other words, the metonymy of reducing humans to goods must be overturned so that we may reactivate the metaphor of exchange and meaningful discourse. In short, African Americans must simultaneously keep a vigil on observing the many ways in which the transgressor has and may attempt to cause them injury as well as continuing to find new and exciting ways to overturn the received injury.

A crisp example of the phenomenon of transgenerational haunting can be found in Carolivia Herron's (1991) novel *Forever Johnnie*. There, she spells out one haunting scenario after another: (1) the females shall be raped by slave masters; the males shall be murdered by slave masters; (2) the males who are not murdered shall be sold away; (3) the males who are neither murdered nor sold away shall marry the females who are not murdered or sold away; (4) in marriage, enslaved males and former slaves shall have revenge over females perceived to have consented to the destruction of males; (5) women and daughters shall therefore be raped over and over again by enslaved men or former slaves.

This is a sequence of appropriative and appositional shifts and transfers where there occurs: (1) the historical presentation of rape and murder in the first instance, (2) appropriation by an ethnic group of a transgressor's cruelty to serve a secondary purpose of revenge, and (3) ossification of a structure of experience that says that victims may heap cruelty that once originated with external transgressors onto their own kind. In transgenerational haunting, then, a concrete staging, a doubling, a reactivation of sedimented historical grievances, a replay, and an extension occur, and it is this transformation that starts the process of losing sight of one's historical or contemporary enemy.

Now, whether or not Europeans or Euro Americans actualize their dominant vision of finding living with others to be unnecessary, I hold that the received hatred can be overturned by African Americans. I hold further that the hospital community, outreach groups, and clinical settings of many kinds can be meaningful laboratories for patients, health professionals, policy makers, and others to negotiate racism and to overturn its destructive consequences. However, regardless of who did what to whom in history, an ethical system of mutual implications must operate in ways which enable us to understand that when one group changes for the better, the whole prospers; when one person grows, he or she grows with the other; when the obligation to grow with the other is grasped as a necessary ethical position, the interests of self and other are yoked.

B. Conceptual Strategy: Linking Basic Assumptions to Tactical Community Action

Here, clinicians must make a motivational shift from conceptualizing their grasp of the nuances of history to a sense of history, and they must do so in ways that link history to the potential for change in our communities. Here concepts like introjection with the aggressor (Ferenczi, 1924) or identification with the aggressor (Anna Freud, 1946) are, in my view, incomplete, although they are correct in their rightful places in psychoanalytic practice. In working with aggrieved communities and pooled communal memories that continue to have destructive impact on the present, a description of shared communal injury must include: (1) the fact of historical injury; (2) the potential for transformation of that history; and (3) a constant reminder that each person, family, or ethnic group must know the motivation behind the historical injury caused by the transgressor.

I want to suggest that the fact of history has an urgency; it cries out for recognition and meaning. The will to transform the injury of history is a necessary volitional process with slippages because breaking away from bondage requires mourning and a related process of self-invention. The historical motivation behind the transgressors' will to hurt, injure, kill, colonize, or extinguish the Other en masse is appropriated as an errand. In another context of describing the phenomenon of transgenerational haunt-ing and its relation to such clinical entities as core gender identity disor-der, anorexia nervosa, and schizophrenia, I (Apprey, 1996b) have drawn attention to a haunting statement by the mother of a transsexual who was treated by Robert Stoller (1968). In the mother's words: "I had died and was already dead but my mother was so busy sending me to the store on errands that she did not notice I was dead." A good metaphor to capture this essence of transgenerational haunting is Auden's phrase where he jux-taposes ships posted on urgent, voluntary errands. I have yet to find an appropriate clinical term that captures the urgency of compelling historical fact, the will to transform the received hatred, and the responsibility that an errand is continuing to be carried out in one form or another. The errand is an abiding one threatening to take root or reluctantly yield to transfor-mation. Invariably! In health or in sickness! The peremptory urges behind repetition are formidable adversaries.

If this motivational shift from history to transformation is not grasped in its tripartite inclusive form, several consequences may befall the clinician. If clinicians emphasize only the urgency of remembering history, subjects, patients, ethnic groups only get angrier. There is, as it were, a repeat of the experience of history in affective form. If clinicians only emphasize the will to change and bypass history, subjects, clients, ethnic groups experi-ence a sense of woundedness once again. They hear the voice of the trans-gressor saying that their history of devastation does not matter. However, by considering the wounds of the living, as it were, together with the will and responsibility to transform the received injury, one gets to transform the toxic errand of extinction, humiliation, massacre, a legacy of ashes, and so on, into a positive errand.

C. Praxis

What do injured communities put into the wound? How may they suture the rupture, the wound of an absence? Appropriating the language of the French phenomenologist Maurice Merleau-Ponty (1983), I would say that the behaviors utilized by injured ethnic groups to fill the gap, to suture the wound, may be described as: (1) syncretic, (2) amovable, and (3) symbolic.

In syncretic behavior, the structure of experience is concrete and is embedded very tightly into the conditions of materiality. Tell an ape that this is a chair to sit on; the ape will most likely use the chair as a chair. Here, the structure of experience is very tightly immersed in the concrete conditions of materiality so that the signification chair as chair is the only expected one.

In contrast to the syncretic, the structure of experience in symbolic behavior suggests that the behavior can be lifted from the conditions of concrete materiality and described independently so that a symbol is both a thing and other than itself. So, if you tell me that a chair is for me to sit on it, I might add other and multiple functions. I can sit on it. In addition, I can hang my coat on the back rest. If this were a glass building and there were fire, I could pick up that same chair, smash a window, and get out of the room.

With regard to amovable behavior, there are degrees of differentiation accompanied by an emergent phantasy life where a phantom of a gloating cynical parent may occupy one's inner world. Here change is not sustained. Change is frowned upon or enacted with tremendous difficulty. For the ancestors of once colonized or enslaved African Americans, the internal assassin looks at his or her progress with contempt.

Why these three categories? The syncretic tells us about incest, murder, direct boundary violations, and other concretely staged acts of grievance or expressions of human desire. For example, "I saved her life, I can sleep with her." One may ask what saving a young woman's life has to do with sexual molestation. Such a syncretic juxtaposition of two unrelated issues can fill the wound of an absence. Here, the immaturity of the adult is reflected in and is concretized in the immaturity of the child when the adult believes the lie that saving a life has something to do with sexually causing a girl, a daughter, or a woman injury which can devastate her for years.

In this situation, the ghost of a slave master turned rapist, the host of a slave who is raped, tortured, or killed, the present-day African American who, as guest houses ancestral figures who are in constant destructive conversation and internal war, are tightly fitted together. In the words of Parveen Adams (1996), a British psychoanalytic scholar on sexual differences, "inside and outside rely on a certain coincidence rather than an opposition" (p. 148). For her, the terms inside and outside are radically implied in each other. She adds: "Within such reasoning the subject, a space of interiority, establishes a relation with the world, a space of exteriority which consists in just the right amount of internalization and externalization for normality to exist and persist" (p. 149). For her the interior and exterior, linked but separate, have a "preordained isomorphism" (p. 149) where the two spaces are invariably already there, already made for each other, yoked and yet separate. In a word, interior and exterior are for the subject who is tied to a syncretic way of behaving, consciousness syntonic. I hold that the ghost, the host, and the guest are now one agent who is today urgently striving to repeat historical injury, choosing an inappropriate object to attack during the repetition, and haphazardly repeating the errand toward extinction or haphazardly recreating a wayward child.

In the case of amovable behavior, there is a new signification where there are partial shifts with particular meanings. For example, a woman whose conduct-disordered child I successfully treated said to me: "You treated my child and I thank you. I am not your patient. I will see a psychiatrist for medication for my Tourette's syndrome." Six months later, I heard over the radio that she had been dismissed by her college for harassing her students. Now, instead of us dealing with and treating the consequences of incest by her father, the whole community was dealing with who causes whom injury, what constitutes harassment, and what happens when a tenured college professor is on trial.

Here the slave master has been internalized as an internal saboteur, an internal assassin, one who kills off the subject's will to recovery and constantly and cynically gloats at that subject's failures. Here any potential success alternates with self-destructive activity. The phantom of an assassin reigns in this domain. Witness the effort of patients who wish to recover in treatment but miss sessions whenever progress is implied or mentioned in relation to their current behavior. The phantom demands that extinction in one form or another be avidly pursued. That phantom is merciless in demanding a destruction that is already mandated. What is left to be done is for the subject to choose his or her form of self-destruction.

In contrast, symbolic behaviors have given the internal assassin a decent burial, knowing that the phantom is part of the self and cognizant that the ghost may return if one is not vigilant or resilient. Adams might suggest here that the internal object of the assassin may be "emptied out." To the notion of "emptied out," I would prefer the notion that the agency of the internal assassin is deferred, suspended or detoxified without any suggestion that the emptying out is final.

These three behavioral practices of syncretic, amovable, and symbolic categories are phenomenological. They are a starting point and are not meant to be exhaustive or frozen into fixed compartments. After all, there is no behavior that never descends below the symbolic level and no behavior that never rises above the syncretic level.

Now that we are familiar with the syncretic, amovable, and symbolic structures of behavior and what they stand for, let me suggest an extended use of these categories to infuse clinical thought in the creative arts and expressive therapies: art therapy, dance and movement therapies, drama therapy, horticultural therapy, music therapy, poetry therapy, psychodrama, and other modalities of intervention. In order to operationalize the structures of experience in the creative arts and expressive therapies, we may conceptualize transgenerational haunting as continuous and yet discontinuous. It is continuous only in the sense that each generation is linked to another biologically and in terms of ego and/or superego identifications. However, the relationship between one generation and another is discontinuous with decisive ruptures, appropriations, and transformations.

Accordingly, one generation of traumatized people may be so close to a trauma that they may choose to never speak about it to their children. Nevertheless, choosing to be silent does not mean that the next generation will not experience in uncanny ways the experience of the previous one. The generation that is "frozen" with the trauma will "inject" messages, precepts, and projects or mandates into the next one which, in turn, may stage or enact in another way the experience of the previous one. The frozen generation, then, may choose to communicate with a syncretic structure of behavior. The next may represent the syncretic presentation of the trauma in an amovable form. In short, one may house in one generation the phantom of another generation. With treatment, a third generation may transform the amovable into a symbolic structure of behavior where there are choices, flexible modes of situating oneself in the world and multiple ways of overturning the received "poison" of history, as it were.

Returning to the "transgressor" who says, "I saved her life when she was a child and so I felt I could sleep with her," let us examine how the syncretic may move to the amovable. A horrified clinician will mostly hear the primitive thinking associated with this case of incest. A moral stance will mostly allow a clinician to see the situation as a crime. However, a disciplined phenomenologist who is no less moral or ethical will be able to capture a multiplicity of potential meanings in this act of incest. For example, capturing the many sides of the subject's naive and syncretic thought, we can hear the following:

> Many years ago, I was terrified that she would die. In fact, I already gave her up "for dead." It dawned on me that I could resuscitate her. I did, and fortunately she lived. She was six years old at the time. Eight years later, when she was fourteen, I just did it, not thinking anything about it. Now, when I look back, it does not seem right.

A time warp collapsed two-time frames of the time of saving her life, and the time of incest into a syncretic structure of behavior. The 14-year-old would soon have three more children with her much older brother-in-law and psychological father. Now an adult, she was haunted by profound superego anxiety in an amovable structure of behavior. It was up to her teenage daughter whom I subsequently treated to overturn the received historical injury in a symbolic way.

There is the potential to transform structures of behavior transgenerationally. In the creative arts and expressive therapies, various opportunities for dramatizing and transforming the storied texts of trauma exist. In art therapy, narratives of who one is, where one is, and where one sees oneself as going in life can be the subject of drawing, painting, and sculpting. Various degrees of transformation are potentially there to be grasped and negotiated. In dance therapy, a clinician can explore with a client where in one's body the traumatic pain is stored or how it is that a patient walks as if she does not own her own body. In psychodrama and/or in drama therapy, life themes can be portrayed, staged, enacted, extended, and transformed in the context of negotiating how one can be both separate from and yoked to one's family. Horticultural therapies can use plants to indicate how one plant gives life to another.

There are many clinical methods for understanding and transforming the impact of historical trauma and reinventing the self in the clinical process. However, the approach advocated here requires that regardless of what clinical method of intervention is chosen, a particular strand must run through the process of treatment to endure durable and meaningful change. This strand must run through psychoanalysis, creative, and expressive arts therapies as well as many forms of intervention in aggrieved communities. The strand includes understanding human suffering, the way that particular suffering is mentalized by the victimized group and subsequently reenacted by generations to come. In technical terms there must first be many profiles of understanding of the historical injury. Then there must be an understanding of how the aggrieved community has stored in their communal memory those psychological hurts, those feelings of humiliation, and changing historical accounts of the actual injuries. Subsequently those sedimentations of historical grievances are enacted within the transference in the clinical situation where the grievances are not only staged, but restaged, distorted, or extended. Then comes the most decisive obligation the clinician has towards the analysand, patient, client, or community that is attempting to transform itself. That decisive obligation is to extract the errand or ambush towards extinction and to undergo the unpleasant drudgery of constantly engaging the mandate to die or destroy oneself in order to find new and more flexible forms of adaptation. In short, to know death is to put it back where it belongs in history as well as knowing how victims may unconsciously house so much bitterness that they may uncannily carry out their own extinction without knowing it and without the assistance of their historical enemy.

It is my view that the reactivation, staging, and extension of historical grievances typically present themselves phenomenologically in terms of syncretic, amovable, and symbolic structures of behavior. Many disciplines can operationalize these distinctions in order to facilitate transformation and reinvention of selves.

In terms of representative forms of community intervention, let us now abandon temporarily the three phenomenological categories of syncretic, amovable, and symbolic that can be helpful with individual interventions in order to consider three types of community interventions: (1) psychopolitical dialogues between community factions in order to reduce tensions or to solve a particular problem, (2) secondary prevention to treat ailments in the community, and (3) primary prevention.

First, I want to draw attention to subgroups within ethnic groups that only want to remember the grievances of the ethnic group. They tend to be two dimensional. They only want to remember. When they act, they typically break the law and end up directly ambushing themselves towards their own demise. Gangs of a particularly virulent kind belong to this category. Some political activists belong to this group when they are two dimensional in focus. They act as the archivists of the sins perpetrated upon them as an ethnic group.

To the extent that these groups act as the archivists of the hurts perpetrated on their ethnic group I do not wish to dismiss them. Rather, when they are not breaking the law, I envisage dialogue between these groups and representatives of the community. I have elsewhere described this process in the context of my work in conflict resolution with Estonia and its Russian population (Apprey, 1996c, 1997a, 1997b).

Here, I shall briefly allude to a less inflammatory context than work with gangs in which, let us say, an urban police department and a group of African American ministers or other civic leaders may attempt a dialogue in order to promote reconciliation or to discover healthier means of coexistence. I shall limit myself to two parties in conflict in this methodology.

Some basic assumptions guide this methodology:

Corollary 1: In the field of conflict resolution, any conception of the Other as fixed or absolute dangerously lends itself to the readiness to dehumanize the Other.

Corollary 2: The facile notion that "we are one blood" is not a helpful solution because it poses a threat to a much-needed sense of self stability and differentiation.

Corollary 3: Of even greater threat to participant groups in conflict is any notion of the self as changing or relative because a precipitous readiness to change poses a threat to a group's identity.

Self as agency is therefore an approximation, the Other as absolute a misnomer, but when Self and Other engage in a process of resolution of a conflict, a new opportunity opens up, fostering a measured exchange of representations of Self and Other. When the process is well modulated by the facilitators, four waystations typically emerge: (1) polarization where each side needs to define itself while demonizing the Other; (2) differentiation within each side, while recognizing the multiplicity of positions in each separate group; (3) the crossing of mental borders where each side engages the Other in a metaphor driven and meaningful dialogue, replacing old concrete passions with a new order of designations to which all parties can relate, typically a new order of designation propelled by an ethic of responsibility for each side; (4) ethical statements become grounded when participant groups join forces to create concrete and mutually beneficial projects.

Second, community projects that try to tackle the problems of drug addiction and teenage pregnancy are paradigmatic forms of intervention that deal with not-so-sudden death, indirect forms of destroying families and communities. There are also very helpful official community interventions such as community policing and other forms of constructive collaboration between citizens and the law. These belong to the area of secondary prevention. Here, harm has already been done. We want to treat and or prevent further injury.

Third, in the area of primary prevention where no obvious harm has as yet been done, I want to draw attention to those community interventions that continue to renew individuals, families, and communities. Such interventions are multidimensional in purpose. For example, Saturday academies for youth in African American communities teach students precepts for living, cognitive skills, leadership skills, and so on and so forth. The emphasis here is on increasing the capacity to renew oneself by having greater options in any given situation as well as having the resilience to bounce back after mental or physical injury.

Addendum

A Note on the Poisoning of Nostalgia

Returning now to the phenomenological categories of syncretic, amovable and the symbolic, I want to suggest that the predominantly extrapsychic impulse toward destruction of self and/or others kills off genuine nostalgia for Africa as a motherland. Likewise, the largely intrapsychic destruction of progress in oneself in the case of amovable structures of experience suggests that genuine nostalgia is not an object of preoccupation. Rather, the syncretic and amovable structures of experience lend themselves to confusion, idealization or denigration. However, the capacity for genuine nostalgia is available to those symbolic structures of experience where there is a multiplicity of and flexibility in profiles of one's cathexis of history. Subjects who operate with flexible symbolic structures do not need to visit Africa in order to feel at home in America. They do not need to idealize or denigrate Africa or America. Rather, they are able to visit Africa when they can and enjoy the novelty of the experience with a wide range of thoughts, feelings, and sensations without bondage to a particular subjectivity of experience. This subject of nostalgia requires further elaboration in another work where it can receive the full attention it deserves. Nevertheless, we have an outline and a schema here to begin that expatiation.

References

Adams, P. (1996). *The Emptiness of the Image: Psychoanalysis and Sexual Differences*. London & New York: Routledge.

Apprey, M. (1996a). Broken lines, public memory, absent memory: Jewish and African Americans coming to terms with racism. *Mind and Human Interaction*, 7(3): 139–149.

Apprey, M. (1996b). *Phenomenology of Transgenerational Haunting: Subjects in Apposition, Subjects on Urgent/Voluntary Errands*. Ann Arbor, MI: U.M.I. Research Collections.

Apprey, M. (1996c). Heuristic steps for negotiating ethnonational conflicts: Vignettes from Estonia. *New Literary History*, 27(2): 199–212.

Apprey, M. (1997a). Alterity as process in the resolution of ethnonational conflicts: The case of Estonia. *Journal for the Psychoanalysis of Culture and Society*, 2(2): 121–128.

Apprey, M. (1997b). *Ethnonational Conflict Resolution between Estonia and Its Russians: A System of Mutual Implications*. Ann Arbor, MI: U.M.I. Research Collections.

Ferenczi, S. (1924). *Thalassa: Theory of Genitality*. New York: Psychoanalytic Quarterly.

Freud, A. (1946). *The Ego and the Mechanisms of Defense*. New York: International Universities Press.

Herron, C. (1991). *Forever Jonnie*. New York: Random House.

Lyotard, J. F. (1991). *Phenomenology*. Albany, NY: State University of New York Press.

Merleau-Ponty, M. (1983). *The Structure of Behavior*. Pittsburgh, PA: Duquesne University Press.

Miller, J. H. (1992). *Ariadne's Thread: Story Lines*. New Haven, CT: Yale University Press.

Stoller, R. J. (1968). *Sex and Gender*. New York: Aronson.

Todorov, T. (1993). *On Human Diversity*. Boston: Harvard University Press.

Chapter 8

A Pluperfect Errand

A Turbulent Return to Beginnings in the Transgenerational Transmission of Destructive Aggression[1]

Introduction: The Operational Format of the Chapter

We begin in Part A with the definition of unconscious transgenerational transmission of destruction aggression in psychoanalysis. The overdetermined meanings of the word "errand" are infused with this account of transmission. The idea of an errand suggests that there is a subject that *urgently* transmits a toxic infusion and an object that *voluntarily* receives it. There is agency, to be sure, but what is the relation of subject to object? It is suggested that subject and object change places. A literary representation in the form of a film, *Incendies* (Denis Villeneuve, Canada/France, 2010), is provided to contextualize this inquiry and to expand our understanding of the trajectory from self to other and then back to the self as that who returns to oneself or to representations of beginnings.

In Part B, a second literary representation in the form of a play, *Forests*, by the same author, Wadji Mouawad (2009b), is used to provide a symbolic reconfiguration and a suture for the gap in the transgenerational rupture.

In Part C, we recognize that while the idea that self returns to self is sufficiently represented, there is something missing. What is conspicuous by its absence is that there are secrets that are injected by anterior or ancestral objects in the transmission of destructive aggression. These secrets are housed in the mental representation of the subject's inside mother and in particular compartments, compartments that both protect and can fatally confine the subject. A psychoanalytic account that discusses secrets and sincerity and the descent of the subject that carries secrets into the deeper recesses of our minds must be added to the idea of the pluperfect errand.

DOI: 10.4324/9781003389026-9

The work of the post-Kleinian "phenomenologist" Donald Meltzer on the "claustrum" (1992) is our best fit here.

Part A: Transgenerational Transmission and Deadly Errands

I: Dreams of Urgent Voluntary Errands

The phenomenon of transgenerational transmission of destructive aggression is increasingly receiving due attention from psychoanalysts (Abraham, 1988; Apprey, 1992, 1993, 2003, and 2006; Volkan, 2004; Faimberg, 2005). Abraham (1988) gave us the idea of the phantom as a metapsychological construct when he linked family secrets to *unconsciously embedded and entombed conflicts* in subsequent generations. Apprey (1992, 1993, 2003, and 2006) takes Freud's instinct theory and radicalizes that into a transgenerational object relations theory for understanding the residual impact of slavery as well as the implications for clinical psychoanalytic practice. Faimberg (2005) used Freud's view that "the ego is not a master in its own house" (Freud, 1917, p. 143) to formulate her technique of listening to narcissistic links between generations. Volkan (2004) articulated his view of actualized unconscious fantasies that accrue from childhood traumas and associated ego restrictions that cause adults to experience or repeat derivatives as though they were real in adult life. These and other accounts of transgenerational transmission are horizontal [sic] and not interchangeable. They are horizontal in the sense that they all give us different but related accounts of how sedimentations of history are reactivated and come to serve new and contemporary purposes (Apprey, 2006). In all my accounts of transgenerational transmission of destructive aggression (1992, 2006), I have emphasized that tension between urgently and unconsciously infused aggression from the external world, on the one hand, and unconsciously appropriated toxic intrusions that I have come to call *dreams of urgent voluntary errands*.

II: Errands

"Errand" here speaks to the idea that there is someone's intentionality that will come or has come to be made one's own. It is central to the understanding of the way the word "errand" is used here that we look at the multiple implications of its meaning. Implicated here in the psychological use of the word "errand" is a composite idea that there is a potential *"error,"* a *"wandering away,"* a *"mistake,"* and a *"mandate"* to be carried out *by the subject for an internal object*. The result is the following ten-fold taxonomy.

1 Something is *injected* from an *anterior source*.
2 That hitherto injected pro-ject [sic] is *housed* in a hospitable place for storage for an indeterminate time.
3 That same something is now *suspended* and *its transfer is deferred*.
4 That something of a project that is stored in this time warp carries *a mandate for an errand* to be carried out.
5 The mandate is accommodated with an *urgent voluntary reception*.
6 The *subject awaits a suitable new object to reawaken the project so that the self-same project or a derivative project can return to a public space* away from the haunt, as it were.
7 By this time the *subject shall have lost sight of who originally sent whom*.
8 *Active and passive have by now become interchangeable.*
9 A *middle voice happening emerges that is neither entirely active nor entirely passive, and* it does so *in an invisible and inaudible way*.
10 Through a middle-voiced happening, the subject returns to itself or to some concrete presentation of beginnings.

Who is the subject that returns to itself or to concrete and unrepresented beginnings? In order to answer this question, let us turn to Claude Romano (2009), a recent French phenomenologist.

III: The Return of the Subject to Oneself

Whereas the subject in psychoanalysis encounters multiple truths, the subject in Descartes (1909) is realized through its engagement with truth. Whereas in Husserl (1977), the father of phenomenology, the researcher describes and deepens that description of the phenomenon under study until that researcher shall have arrived at an intersubjective constitution for the subject whose phenomenal and experiential world is being inter-rogated, the subject in Claude Romano is one who comes to oneself *(adv-enant)*. In Romano (2009), that return to oneself takes place in the middle space between self and other, and these events are reconfigured so that events become represented as middle voiced happenings. In the process of reconfiguring events into representations, events in Romano become what he calls *eventials* [sic]. Parenthetically, I must add that he italicizes new words like "advenant" and "evential" for emphasis throughout his work so that we can grasp the decisive reconfiguration of the mental world that he is addressing.

Romano (2009), then, distinguishes between two types of events. When events happen they actualize a possibility that is already present in the world, like lightning. On the other hand, *events as evential* overturn existing possibilities and in so doing *reconfigure the world.* In Romano's words, in the *evential reconfiguration*

> the one who understands is strictly implicated in the very act of understanding: I can understand an event as being addressed to me only if I am myself in play in the possibilities it assigns to me [me destine] and through which it makes history by opening a destiny for me.
>
> (2009, p. 30)

In my view, *there is a system of mutual implications between the event as fact for the one to whom the concrete event happens and the one who re-shapes what that event does to him or her and determines what that event means.*

In a bald summary of Romano's phenomenology of the *evential*, four shifts show themselves. I shall summarize these four shifts that give themselves.

1   During the reconfiguration of the subject's world, a *metamorphosis that is impossible to date* takes place. Once an event is brought about, *it is already too late.* We are therefore never contemporaries of the actualization of the event.
2   We can experience it *when an event has already taken place*, and this is why, says Romano, *an event* in the eventness happens only *according to the secrets of its latency.*
3   Accordingly, an event is not the datable fact of the meeting of two beings but rather that which lies in reserve in this meeting *and* which *gives it its future loading.*
4   The subject therefore is *an advenant* that comes *back to oneself.* The subject that returns to a prior latency shall have come back to oneself after revealing *the secret that lies or has lain in reserve.*

How, then, are we to understand in a palpable way a metamorphosis of an event that is not datable? How are we to understand how we go back to secrets of human existence that both take us back and lie in wait for us?

In psychoanalysis we know the story of Oedipus. There is, however, an equally powerful modern-day Sophoclean story, written by Wadji Mouawad, an award-winning Canadian playwright and director. His film *Incendies* (2010) was nominated for an Oscar in 2010 and has won other prestigious awards. It was translated into English by Linda Gaboriau as *Scorched* (2009a). This is one powerful story that ought to get the attention of every psychoanalyst. I shall use it to launch the term *pluperfect errand of the unconscious in transgenerational haunting*. It is an errand because it lies in reserve waiting to happen. We have here an exquisite representation of *a pluperfect errand, a parental project that has already happened but was only lying in wait for its messenger(s)*, in Wadji Mouawad's *Incendies*.

IV: Incendies *and Deadly Errands*

Nawal Marwal gives birth to her twins, Jeanne and Simon. Upon her death, her now-grown twins attend a reading of *their mother's will*. In her last testament, Jeanne must deliver a letter to her father. In this context, a will is both a testament and a demand: a witnessing and a project. Simon must deliver a letter to *a* lost brother of whom the twins had been unaware. Trails provide incremental details until each sibling discovers the person each has been sent to find.

Now we must pause to either watch the film, *Incendies* (2010), or read the book, *Scorched* (2009a), and/or proceed with my rendition.

I shall now use four movements, albeit arbitrarily chosen to illustrate what I mean by *the pluperfect latency of the unconscious* in transgenerational haunting. I shall use four rubrics to indicate the movements: (1) the *reception* of the deadly errand, (2) the *aggressive incursion* into the mental world of the twins, (3) the *appropriation* of the errand, and (4) the tumultuous return to oneself: a restitution of a kind.

(1) The Reception of the Errand

To Janine, her mother mandates the following: "this envelope is for . . . your father and Simon's. Find him and give him this envelope" (p. 8). As disturbing as the errand is for each offspring, the mandate has a suitable home. *They feel obligated to carry out a wish they may not refuse.* It feels *urgent*. How does the urgent mandate become *voluntary*?

(2) The Aggressive Incursion of the Mandate to Render It Voluntary

The mother's errand is soon appropriated. Janine says to her brother: "*I am going to find this father of ours, and if I find him, if he is alive, I'll give him the envelope. I'm not doing it for her; I am doing it for myself.* And for you. For the future" (p. 69; italics added). Once their mother's *urgent* errand is appropriated it becomes *voluntary*, and in effect, it becomes a new errand to find "Mama." Accordingly, Janine says to Simon: "We have to find her past, her life during all those years she hid from us. . . . The hole I am about to tumble into, the hole I am already slipping into, is that of her silence" (p. 69).

(3) The Aggressive Injection

The brother that Simon is looking for is *already* looking for his mother. The father Janine is looking for is *already* looking for his mother. How is he looking for his mother? In wartime, a turbulent time telecast as the Lebanese civil war in *Incendies*, the child looking for his mother is orphaned, lost. When civil war strikes, the orphanage that houses the lost child is decimated. But he falls into the hands of the enemy that blows up the orphanage. He is spared because the enemy sees something in him. The enemies revel in his marksmanship and keep him and treat him as one of their own. He swears in his turn that the world will come to know him for his marksmanship. That capability of becoming the most accomplished marksman is how his mother will come to hear of him and thereby know him. On his mother's part, she assassinates a nationalist leader and is jailed, but her life is spared. Who becomes her jail guard? Her own son, unbeknownst to her.

As Romano tells us, eventials are not datable. Their secrets lie in reserve. Mother and jailor son look for each other. *Their search has already happened. They have already found each other.* In jail, in the domain of aggression "no one ever spoke her name. She was simply the woman who sings, number seventy two. . . . The woman who assassinated the paramilitary leader. . . . All her friends were captured and killed. Only the one who sings survived" (p. 92). How does she survive? Her son has a new identity, Abou Tarek. He handles her in jail.

> The night when Abou Tarek raped her, *we could not tell their voices apart.* . . . And inevitably she got pregnant. . . . He searched for his mother; he found her but did not recognize her. She searched for her son, she soon found him, and didn't recognize him. He didn't kill her, because she sang, and he liked her voice.
>
> (p. 99; italics added)

A system of mutual implications follows: "Abou Tarek tortured [his] mother, and [his] mother was tortured by her son and the son raped his mother. The son is the father of his brother and sister" (p. 99).

(4) Restitution as a Tumultuous Return to Oneself

Nawal speaks to her daughter and son, Janine and Simon, in a way that is haunting and does point to restitution as a tumultuous return to oneself as follows: "Where does your story begin? At your birth? Then it begins in horror. At your father's birth? Then it is a beautiful love story. Perhaps we will discover that *his love story has roots in violence and rape.* And in turn, *the brute and the rapist had his origin in love*" (p. 134, italics added).

What kept the mother from telling her story before?

> *"There are truths that can only be revealed when they have been discovered."*
>
> (p. 134; emphasis added)

V: The Pluperfect Errand That Lies Waiting to Be Discovered

When truths can only be told or revealed when they have *already* been discovered, we are in the realm of *a pluperfect latency.* It is quite apt to use Wadji Mouawad's own words in his own introduction to his next play, *Forests* (2009b), to put an exclamation mark on a pluperfect latency as a phenomenal idea that shapes how stories come to him, how he receives what gives itself as a story to him, how a narrative spots him so that he does not have to invent it. He writes: "Events often catch us unaware.

They have been determined; *they have already come and gone by the time we realize it*. We can no longer see them or study them, because time has taken us forward" (Mouawad, 2009b, p. iii; emphasis added). What is left after the events' phenomenal appearance? "All that is left is the shock of their appearance, their entrance into the visible. Our visible" (Mouawad, 2009b, p. iii).

Part B: Transgenerational Transmission and the Reconfiguration of Pluperfect Errands

The film *Incendies* (2010) and its play, *Scorched* (2009a), have given us a return of the subject to oneself, the subject that Romano calls *advenant*. In a restitutive move, each twin in *Scorched* has now come to experience a return to beginnings and what I would like to call the tumultuous return to oneself, but *an expanded orbit of oneself*. Who inhabits that orbit? Each self is *self as child of one's mother*, to be sure. Each son or daughter has a sibling for a father. Now Janine must accommodate that incest which has already taken place. To reiterate, she is a product of incest; she has a brother for her father. Simon must likewise add a new structure of experience to his representational word. He is his brother's son. Their discoveries or rediscoveries constitute a dead end: an aporia. An aporetic return hitherto created by the peremptory, instinctual, or Sophoclean Oedipal return must now be overturned. In *Forests* (2009b), we have the representation of an answer to the aporia.

Forest *and an Artistic and Symbolic Transformation*

If *Incendies* masterfully depicts a deadly pluperfect errand, the play *Forests* provides a symbolic depiction of the interruption of deadliness and a possibility for transformation of transgenerationally transmitted toxic mandates. Earlier, we used four movements to indicate (1) the reception of the deadly errand, (2) the aggressive injection, (3) the appropriation, and (4) the disturbing return to oneself. Now we can use the text of *Forest* to give us a literary representation of the trajectory of the pluperfect errand and its interruption. First, a pluperfect latency that lies in reserve, waiting to happen, is depicted. Second, an *aporia*, a dead end, is depicted. Third, the wound caused by the aporia undergoes a *suture*. Finally, *generativity is restored* so that a new generation may not repeat the mandate to destroy itself or future generations to follow.

Forest *and the Text of the Pluperfect Latency That Lies in Reserve, Waiting to Happen*

Alexandre, a father, along with his second wife, Mathilde, tells his son, Albert, that he wants him to keep his and Mathilde's assets and in turn pass them on to the next generation of children and their grandchildren. Albert is not impressed. He observes his father's ardent wish to make him into a man who resembles him and speaks to the panic that follows his father's demand inside him as a son of his father. Albert, as son, notices further-more that every son wants to climb up to his father, "but some fathers climb to such unimaginable heights for fear of being equaled, while con-tinuing to insist upon it" (Mouawad, 2009b, p. 79). Albert wants to shatter his father's hopes, shatter his father's name, honor, and reputation "with-out disappearing, without ceasing to exist" (p. 79).

Accordingly, he wants to announce to his father that he intends to get married to Odette against his father's will, and does. He makes his announcement and does marry her in order to free himself from his father. The problem is that his father Alexandre has *already* met Odette.

Alexandre has already impregnated Odette. It is *already* too late for Albert, the son, to build a new life free of his father's influence. *Incest has already con-fused [sic] the generations.*

Albert's wife, Odette, will deliver twins after a vain effort to kill the children in her womb. Now Albert's son, Jérémie, will be his brother, and Albert's daughter, Hélène, will be his sister.

Jérémie and Hélène, twins and the product of incest, repeat the pluperfect latency that lies in reserve, waiting to happen. Anxious to break out of it, Jérémie tells his twin sister that he cannot stand the thought of their father touching her; she is his sister. He wants them to leave. "We've been living in this forest since we were born and we are slowly going crazy, nuts, insane, loony, and raving mad. His dream is devouring us. It's *his dream,* Hélène, *not ours*" (Mouawad, 2009b, p. 108; emphasis added). The problem is that Albert's dream to multiply across generations has *already* happened. Albert has *already* confused the generations. Albert has already seduced Hélène.

Hélène is his daughter by social convention, his sister biologically. Out-raged by Albert's seduction of Hélène, Jérémie kills Albert and, in rage and outrage, drives "his sex into his sister's body" (p. 117). Whose child would be the product of Albert's and now Jérémie's sexual and assaultive intrusion? We are left with a secret. Léonie and an unnamed son are now born into confusion.

What is critical under the rubric of a pluperfect latency that lies in reserve is that in *Forests, every new generation that tries to free itself from its forebears finds itself ambushed into a prior latency that cannot be reversed*. An aporia ensues.

Textual Depiction of Aporia and the Textual Depiction of Suture

Léonie, another product of violent incest, gives birth to Ludivine. This time, Ludivine is a hermaphrodite who cannot conceive a child. A condition of hermaphroditism comes to represent the aporia of a dead end for the generations. How would the dead end be reconfigured so that growth through subsequent generations may not be foreclosed?

Ludivine cannot bear a child. Her friendship with a Jewish woman, Sarah Cohen, opens the door for the textual representation of a suture. Under persecution, Sarah Cohen faces the threat of death during the Jewish holocaust. Ludivine *exchanges* her name and identity with Sarah Cohen's. Why? "You can bring children into the world, but all I can do is give my life, and who would I rather give it up for than you?" (Mouawad, 2009b, p. 146). Ludivine, taken away as though she were Sarah Cohen, has her skull crushed with the blows of a hammer. The friendship between Sarah Cohen and Ludivine is deep enough that Sarah Cohen's child, Luce, believes she is Ludivine's daughter: "A life saved, a life lost, a life given" (p. 147). The suture that links the generations operates at two levels: a material and a functional level.

At the *material* level, Mouawad's account of the continuation of the generations occurs in the following way. Two generations later, Ludivine mysteriously leaves a trace of herself in the body of Sarah's descendants: "a bone floating in the middle of a mind" (p. 151), in the mind of Luce's daughter, Aimee. At the *functional* level, a deep friendship makes Luce as much Ludivine's daughter as she is Sarah Cohen's. Materially, a remnant of Ludivine's crushed skull, a skull crushed by the Nazis, now lies in Luce's daughter's mind. Functionally, friendship makes the generativity of the generations possible.

Restoration of Generativity

Ludivine and Sarah Cohen represent a combined figure of a mother for Luce. Luce's daughter, Aimée, inhabits a piece of bone that lodges just as much in her mind as it does in Ludivine's mind. Aimée gives birth to Loup. Loup grows up initially believing that the thread of the past condemns her and all that came before. Upon her mother's death and upon grasping the meaning of generational continuity and, in particular, the impact of the suturing effect of friendship, Loup has this to say: "I used to believe I was bound by blood to my ancestor's. I have discovered that I am bound by my promises, to the promises you made to each other, promises you kept. A life saved, a life lost, a live given" (p. 155).

To operationalize her grasp of the tie that binds, she will repeat the name of the women that came before her—"Odette, Hélène, Léonie, Ludivine, Sarah, Luce, Aimée, and Loup like a promise kept forever" (p. 155). To the next generation "I will repeat it in turn to the girl who will come after me yet to be born" (p. 156).

Ludivine was the last to be born to the Keller name—Alexandre, Albert and Odette, Jérémie and Hélène and Léonie, and finally Ludivine. Then there was a rupture. Ludivine, as a hermaphrodite, cannot bear children. The Cohens followed. The coming together of the two names Keller and Cohen speaks to deeper possibilities for a generational continuity that transcends the limits of biology.

Part C: A Psychoanalytic Turn

In *Incendies* (2010) and *Scorched* (2009a), we have a depiction of urgent voluntary errands. In *Forests*, we have an account of destructive errands that are overturned and reconfigured into a creative project with a new agency from within rather than a repetition of an inherited project of destructive aggression. Two sides of a pluperfect errand show themselves in *Incendies* (2010) and *Scorched* (2009a), on one side, and *Forests*, on the other. The former ends in a tumult, the latter in the transformation of a heart that promises to foster creative generativity and generosity.

It would seem that we could end here with the idea that the gaps in transgenerational haunting can be sutured and reconfigured in the external world by friendships, personal sacrifice in meaningful relationships, and other non-clinical relationships. To consider the limits of friendships and other external fields of reference, let us turn to psychoanalysis. In his inaugural paper on transgenerational haunting, Nicolas Abraham (1988) indicated that the phantom associated with this phenomenon is an invention of the living. This invention, in his view, objectifies "the gap that the conceal-ment of some loved one's life produced in us" (1988, p. 75).

What haunts, then, are not the dead. Rather, what haunts are those gaps left within us by the secrets of others. In putting forward his theory of psychic retreats, John Steiner (1993) defined a psychic retreat within the context of a clinical relationship as follows: "an area of relative peace and protection from strain when meaningful contact with the analyst is experi-enced as threatening" (1993, p. 1); a place where

> they retreat behind a powerful system of defences which serve as a protective armour or hiding place, and it is sometimes possible to observe how they emerge with great caution like a snail coming out of its shell and retreat once more if contact leads to pain or anxiety.
>
> (1993, p. 1)

Steiner's felicitous term is evocative of an epistemic place, a secret hideout, as it were, whose function is clearly to seek protection from men-tal pain.

Donald Meltzer (1992), in the course of his investigation of claustro-phobic phenomena and modes of entry into the internal mother, published his work on *The Claustrum* when he masterfully depicted the geographi-cal dimensions of the mental apparatus, the compartments of the inside mother and life within each compartment. The portals of entry, for Melt-zer, into the claustrum may be (1) the head, breast, mouth configuration; (2) the genital; or (3) the anal.

Baldly, the subject that inhabits the oral claustrum functions as though there is an illusion of clarity attached to its grandiose wishes. The subject that inhabits the genital claustrum functions as though one has to invariably scheme or counter scheme to oust others from expectation. The inhabitants of the anal compartment are threatened with expulsion, death, boundary-lessness, merger, disappearance, and other modes of non-existence. Sur-vival is thus the only value.

A film discussion on secrets then has to make a distinction between secrecy, in se, and mystification of secrets where there is an elaborate men-tal scheme to lie to conceal a painful secret or to mentalize external fields of reference so that one has to end up in a psychic retreat, or specifically in a particular compartment. The external fields of reference to secrets may be prescriptions or constraints attached to what it means to marry or conceive a child from another religion. Nawal Narwan, the protagonist in *Incendies*, is one who defies the system of constraints and prescriptions of her family and religion and pays dearly for conceiving a child with a Muslim man. The family must hide the "infamy". The road to a tortured life inside and outside leads to brutality and incest. The withdrawal into silence is not so silent. It is a retreat into an anal claustrum where she must survive at all costs.

In Place of a Conclusion

A subject that is haunted in the process of transgenerational transmission of destructive aggression potentially carries a secret. She must undergo an errand. Unfortunately, the errand shall have already taken place. She may urgently carry out the mandate, even if it spells her own demise, and she may voluntarily choose her mode of self-destruction. The virulence of the mandate determines what retreat she organizes to protect herself from mental pain and what portal of entry for her ensconcement into the mental representation of the inside mother must follow.

A film presentation can depict life in the claustrum. Psychoanalytic treatment must facilitate the exit of the subject from the claustrum; the representation of the compartment of the inside mother where the subject retreats for safety but must not stay if she intends to survive and to prosper. These two projects, the artistic representation and the work of psychoanalysis, need each other. They cannot be antinomies. Rather, we must seek complementarities out of their convergent intentionalities.

Note

1 The authors thank Annie Gibson of Playwrights Canada Press for her permission to reprint material from the following sources: Mouawad, W. (2009a). *Scorched.* Translated by L. Gaboriau. Toronto: Playwrights Canada Press, and Mouawad, W. (2009b). *Forests.* Translated by L. Gaboriau. Toronto: Playwrights Canada Press.

References

Abraham, N. (1988). Notes on the phantom. In *The Trials of Psychoanalysis*, ed. F. Meltzer, pp. 75–80. Chicago: University of Chicago Press.
Apprey, M. (1992). Dreams of urgent voluntary errands. *Melanie Klein and Object Relations,* 10(2): 1–29. Reprinted in Apprey, M. & Stein, H. (1993).

Intersubjectivity, Projective Identification and Otherness. Pittsburgh: Duquesne University Press.

Apprey, M. (2003). Repairing history: Reworking transgenerational trauma. In *Hating in the First Person Plural*, ed. D. Moss. New York: The Other Press.

Apprey, M. (2006). Difference and the awakening of wounds in intercultural analysis. *The Psychoanalytic Quarterly*, LXXV(1): 73–94.

Descartes, R. (1909). *Discourse on Method, Vol. XXXIV, Part 1. The Harvard Classics*. New York: P.F. Collier & Son.

Faimberg, H. (2005). *The Telescoping of Generations: Listening to the Narcissistic Links between Generations*. London & New York: Routledge.

Freud, S. (1917). A difficulty in the path of psychoanalysis. In *Standard Edition*, Volume 17. London: Hogarth Press and the Institute of Psychoanalysis.

Husserl, E. (1977). *Cartesian Meditations*. Translated by D. Cairns. The Hague: Martinus Nijhoff (Orig. 1931).

Meltzer, D. (1992). *The Claustrum*. Perth: Clunie Press.

Mouawad, W. (2009a). *Scorched*. Translated by L. Gaboriau. Toronto: Playwrights Canada Press.

Mouawad, W. (2009b). *Forests*. Translated by L. Gaboriau. Toronto: Playwrights Canada Press.

Romano, C. (2009). *Event and World*. New York: Fordham University Press.

Steiner, J. (1993). *Psychic Retreats*. London: Routledge.

Volkan, V. (2004). Actualized unconscious fantasies and therapeutic play in adult analyses. In *Power of Understanding: Essays in Honor of Viekko Tähka*, ed. A. Laine, pp. 119–141. New York, NY: Routledge.

Chapter 9

Three Leitmotifs for Sequencing and Transforming the Process of Transgenerational Transmission of Destructive Aggression

Introduction

Baldly stated, my account of transgenerational transmission of destructive aggression is as follows. A subject renders an archaic preclinical prehistory from the events of history to a sense of history. Subject creates a representational world with that revised history. In psychoanalysis, the analyst takes the command-laden transference, gives the command in that transference wish a new home in the public space of the clinical setting until a resubjectivization in the form of a sublimation by the subject comes to create one's own exit strategy.

This is the first time I have used the word "command" in any of my work on transgenerational transmission of destructive aggression. I have tended to use these words: an unconscious plea or demand in the transference wish in individual work, and in the case of cultural transmission, I have used the words prescriptions and constraints in "communal memory." Now, I am emboldened to add the word "command" to my repertoire. Why?

In Attic Greek, the verb "archein" has two meanings: "to begin"; and "to command." I am indebted to the Italian philosopher Giorgio Agamben (2019) for theorizing the implications of this double meaning in his book *Creation and Anarchy*. Here is my attraction to the duality. One meaning—to begin—*announces* an inaugural starting point. The second meaning—to command—provides an opportunity for a *strategic shift in comprehension of conception*. Accordingly, when Agamben plays with the first lines of St. John's Gospel, "en arche, in the beginning was the logos, the word," and ponders with us what could have happened if that first sentence had been translated as a command to begin the creation of the logos, we see the profundity of the duality of meanings embedded in the Greek word "archein."

DOI: 10.4324/9781003389026-10

Suppose then that we heard the first lines of St. John's Gospel anew: "In the command was the creation of the logos." Here, "to begin" and "to command" are horizonal, but not interchangeable. For Agamben, then, the beginning is already a command, a principle. For me, in this chapter, an explosion of birth, as it were.

I have come to draw inspiration from the way Agamben brings duplicity into a unity—to begin is to command—in order to fill a gap in my account of transgenerational transmission. I have variously written about transgenerational transmission with these phrases: "urgent/voluntary errands," appropriated from the poet W.D. Auden (1927) to rethink my way of addressing how a subject, in mental life, peremptorily takes an infusion from an ancestral mandate and chooses one's own poison; "pluperfect errands" to suggest that by the time a subject comes to awareness of the mission as originarily not-one's-own, the toxic errand shall have already taken place; "subjects in apposition" (Apprey, 1993) to account for the continuous deferral across generations of the toxic posting. I have in mind a catalogue of forms of psychical transmission. To that end, I have expanded Freud's idea of "Nachtraglichkeit" (1895) which until recently had insufficiently been translated as "deferral." In a forthcoming paper on transgenerational transmission, I have used the phrase, "Before a call and its response, there was already a *dislocating errand*" in the title and theorized on the call and dislocated subjects. In the body of the paper, I echo Heidegger's (1962) notion of the source of the call that says: the "call comes from me and yet from beyond me and over me" (p. 320; italics in original). This is a tantalizing hint and incomplete account of a call. Something, en arche, precedes me. I want to know more. Then I am drawn to Marion's (2002) view that the *decentered* subject is saturated and thrown but held at the center. Still, we are at a loss regarding the antecedents of the thrownness and dislocation. Romano's (2009) subject is already thrown into a dislocating saturation but may reconfigure the world.

Now, I can fill a gap at the front end. What was once implicit is now explicit. The posting that was in the errand is now commanded *directly* or *indirectly*. In a *direct* command, the agency of the sub-ject [sic] is explicit. In such an errand, someone calls, another responds, and before them, a commander who enjoins and entrusts something to an Other. Such a commander is akin to the spectral representation of Hamlet's father who, as ghost, a revenant, returns to command Hamlet to avenge his death, a mandate that Hamlet considers apt to execute and by which he stays deliriously haunted: a command pointedly given, a mission conflictedly appropriated. A vengeful deed deferred.

In an *indirect* command-in-an-errand, such as *the hint* in a case referenced in the following, an older child interprets a grandmother's consternation upon seeing "disorder" in his younger brother, a toddler, as his responsible opportunity to create an errand to fulfil. He takes her consternation as his mandated command in-an-errand to do something about a grandmother's perception of a child's disorderly play and thus remove the dis-order [sic] a few years later. We shall return to this subject that misinterprets [sic] grandmother's call and executes her errand.

Three Leitmotifs

Each one of Heidegger's (1962), Marion's (2002), or Romano's (2009) idea of a subject's assignment, as it were, is insufficient for my project. Each one has a place. All three constitute one of the following: a starting point, an intermediate space, and a relative closure in the trajectory of transgenerational transmission.

A *sequencing*, then, shows more promise. To be more precise, a sequencing of (1) Heidegger's subject that experiences the spectral mandate as something that comes from me, beyond me, and over me; (2) Marion's subject as one who experiences one's thrownness in a saturation and is yet held at the center; and (3) Romano's resubjectivizing agent's return, in a three-fold aggregate, provides a phenomenological approximation of my account of transgenerational transmission of destructive aggression. In such a phenomenology, something is *designed*, something is *sustained*, something is *reconfigured* again and again until a resubjectivization in treatment can achieve a sublimation that we may call an exit strategy.

These three transition points constitute what I am dubbing "three leitmotifs," as it were. They announce transition points in the quasi-operatic narratives of transgenerational transmission of destructive aggression. Heide Faimberg, in a personal communication, once said that sometime in the fourth or fifth year of a psychoanalysis, the intrapsychic participants in transgenerational transmission announce themselves more fully. While I agree in principle with that observation, I often meet these intrapsychic participants sooner. I meet them in the history-taking process and in the initial phase of analysis, I watch them appear and reappear in the thick of the transference, and I watch them tamed and transformed toward termination. I shall illustrate with dreams and with little historical or identifiable detail so that we can simply focus on the oneiric markers.

The Inaugural Dreams of Urgent Voluntary Errands; Or, "Something Comes From Me, Beyond Me, and Over Me" (Heidegger)

A man who once accidentally committed a fatal crime and was not punished has now come to treatment, decades later, to come to terms with his crime and to determine what is fueling his current state of mental disrepair. Early in treatment he is showing me how he has hitherto represented the events of history into a sense of history. Accordingly, he shows me this rendition from the events of history to a sense of history when he dreams that he is in jail. The inmates attempt a jailbreak. He has an opportunity to escape. He chooses to stay so that he can assist his prison guards to decorate the outside walls of his prison. This first dream gives him the opportunity to provide more details of his crime that went unpunished and, most importantly, a glimpse of the implicit role his father played in the creation of the cavalier attitude of collecting guns without securing them, an act of omission by a father that indirectly led to a son's commission of the fatal accident. As the treatment alliance deepens, he has dreams that show that the prison walls are melting.

The need to be punished for fulfilling the errand appropriated from grandmother to kill his disorderly sibling became modified. He must create his own prison. Analysis began to disturb his self-imposed confinement. I, a Ghanaian psychoanalyst, entered his dreams as the kind general from Nigeria who was a head of state, a double figure of a man who kills and a gentle custodian of power. After the thick cavity walls melted, he began to reveal the latent errand. Grandmother was concerned that the toddler was so disorderly that he would one day become a violent force in the family. He heard the concern and translated the consternation as her wish to remove disorder. His translation of his grandmother's consternation became his errand to kill his younger brother, albeit in an accident. Now a new and kind "general" could stay alive for him as he reconfigured his world, old and new.

In the Thick of the Transference; or, Subject Is "Saturated" and Yet "Held at the Center" (Marion) by the Transference

In the third year of analysis and in the thick of the transference, he was about to repeat a variation of the crime that had tortured him for decades when I interpreted the "megalomania" (my word in the room, and it was uncharacteristic of me to use big words) that drove him to want to urgently wish to repeat his crime in order to be punished now. He registered a mild protest to my motivated error, punitive interpretation, and countertransference wish to punish him by interpreting the megalomania rather than the motivation behind his penchant to repeat that crime and be freshly punished. The next morning, he returned to his session with these words: "I dreamt that Mount Kenya erupted!" Next, and in the thick of the transference, he appropriately dreamt that I was Hades to whom the dead came to confess their sins. After interpreting his enactment and my unconscious reception of his private wish to be punished, his command-laden transference wish that I receive him, punish him, and witness his suffering emerged fully into a transference neurosis. *In the thick of the transference, then, we travel from Ghana, to Nigeria, to Kenya and, eventually, to hell where he could tell me, a stand-in for Hades, his intrapsychic story.* What will his exit strategy from a psychological experience of hell be?

In Place of a Conclusion

Let us return to Freud to see what we have done with his instinct theory. Freud (1915) wrote that an instinct has a source that is biological. It operates under pressure. It has an aim that could be active or passive. It has an object, that is, the body through which the instinctual aim is fulfilled.

When transgenerational transmission is considered in the light of instinct theory, the source of the peremptory urge becomes more than the body. The source exceeds the body. Ancestors enter the picture. Ancestors slowly and insidiously inject their pre-scripted [sic] mandates. Instead of active and passive aims between a subject and an object, multiple subjects operate in apposition, one after another, and in subsequent generations. Grandmother is an active subject. A father in the next generation is an active subject. The child murderer in yet another generation is still an active subject. Subject and object continue to change places without losing agency until the spectral and ancestral wishes are met and transformed by psychoanalysis. In treatment, the command-in-an-errand [sic] to repeat a death, an injury or self-erasure of one kind or another, can be reconfigured. This process of continuous working through opens the doors for sublimation potential to emerge. Now, *the patient can resubjectivize one's own exit strategy from ensconcement to a gradual process of mental emancipation.*

We can now schematize three key phases in an analysis of transgenerational transmission: unpacking the traces of the command in the haunt, if it is accessible in the history and in the early phase of the analysis, by *gathering transference traits* only; *staying alive with and for the patient* as the patient brings the archaic command fully into the analysis so that we can authentically interpret the wishes in the command; and presiding over the processes of *resubjectivizing the archaic errand into an exit strategy.*

On a final note, I am primarily descriptively constitutive in Husserl's sense of being faithful to the mind of a subject when I preside over a psychoanalytic process and Freudian in the broadest scope of framing and moving forward psychoanalytic processes through subsequent and palpable interpretation.

Description without presupposition, then, precedes empirically palpable and constitutive transference-laden interpretation. When I write retrospectively about human phenomena, I can accommodate Husserl's detractors, like Heidegger, Marion, and Romano, by using some of their projects as proximal and evocative borders, not as thematic structures to interrogate, hence the leitmotifs or musical phrases to demarcate shifting contours in a narrative sequence.

References

Agamben, G. (2019). *Creation and Anarchy*. Stanford, CA: Stanford University Press.

Apprey, M. (1993). Dreams of urgent/voluntary errands and transgenerational haunting in transsexualism. In *Intersubjectivity, Projective Identification and Otherness*, eds. M. Apprey & H. Stein, pp. 102–128. Pittsburgh: Duquesne University Press.

Auden, W. H. (1927). On this island. In *The Major Poets*, ed. C. M. Coffin. New York: Harcourt, Brace and World, Inc., 1954.

Freud, S. (1915). Instincts and their vicissitudes. In *Standard Edition of the Complete Psychological Works of Sigmund Freud*, Volume 14, pp. 109–140. London: Hogarth Press.

Heidegger, M. (1962). *Being and Time*. Translated by J. Maquarrie & E. Robinson. New York: Harper and Rowe.

Marion, J.-L. (2002). *Being Given: Toward a Phenomenology of Givenness*. Palo Alto: Stanford University Press.

Romano, C. (2009). *Event and World*. New York: Fordham University Press.

Chapter 10

Transgenerational Transmission in Psychoanalysis

Dislocating Errands

In the process of psychical *transmission* of destructive aggression from one generation to the next, *who asks what of whom?* The evocative expression of an "errand" suggests that a subject is sent on a *mission,* sent *in error, wanders away,* and *returns home, adversely changed.* A *vocative imperative* is at the heart of a mission. When there is a call from an anterior Other, there must be a response. Before there was an experience of a call and its response, then, *there would be an errand.* Precisely, the subject is preceded by the self-same subject's constituted and appropriated mandate from an anterior object. To upend an aberrant errand, a subject must reconfigure a *posted* imperative, ever altering, again and again, the call and summons of an alien and unwelcome *guest* turned *host.* Otherwise, the dissonant and unwelcome guest turned host may transform the naïve subject into a *ghost, a revenant* that disappears and returns to haunt the subject.

Thanks to the new and public space in the clinical setting, the entity that listens to the sub-ject [sic] will come to know that reception and perception of an errand is communalized in ways where there is a constant *alteration, revision,* and *co-creation of meanings* of the received and perceived phenomenon through *reciprocal connection* and *reciprocal correction.* When subject's experiential acquisitions enter that clinical setting, a resolute *upending* of a retrogressive descent toward death may occur. Hence, the meaning of staying alive for an Other who is otherwise *dislocated,* thrown, posted into a transgenerational spiral, toward death. A toxic errand is thus potentially aborted in that new space where a new relationship for resubjectivizing and sublimating the unwanted mandate happens. *Resubjectivizing the injected errand* becomes *the exit strategy* so that positive change is now conceivable.

DOI: 10.4324/9781003389026-11

Introduction

In clinical work, we differentiate between *historical reality* and *psychic reality*, between the *events of history* and the *psychological appropriation of aspects of that history* because they address different motivations, meanings, and clinical procedures. In our hurry to arrive at meanings, clinicians tend to take precipitous leaps from their initial grasp of the *events of history* to their articulation of a meaningful *sense of history*. As a result, the sense of *turmoil, in se*, of the subject, especially by the turbulence of trauma, in that historical period, is not sufficiently interrogated or articulated in either the diagnostic phase or early in the treatment phase. In haste, we proceed to interpretation without standing still with the patient, without fully grasping the concrete materiality, visceral memory, or blood-churning *vital* essence of the phenomenology of the historical narratives themselves. Let us provisionally call this tumult *a dislocation*.

Gaston Bachelard (1939/1979), the French physical chemist turned aesthetician, addressed a similar problem of precipitous leaps, in psychoanalysis, broadly conceived in his reveries on dreams, fire, air, water, and earth, on one hand, and literary symbolism, on the other. He wrote quite eloquently as follows:

> Literary symbolism and *the* symbolism that is Freud's, such as they are executed in classical symbolism and normal dreamwork, are only mutilated examples of the symbolizing powers active in nature. Both represent an expression that has been arrested too soon. They remain substitutes for a substance or person that desert evolution, syntheses named too quickly, desires uttered too soon.
>
> (p. 31; emphasis in original)

"Substitutes . . . that desert evolution" is the key phrase here. His solution? "A new poetry and a new psychology that might describe the soul as it is being formed, language in bloom, must give up definite symbols or images learned merely and *return to vital impulses* and primitive poetry" (p. 31; emphasis added). What is so special about returning to the concreteness, materiality, the physicality of *vital impulses*?

In order to get a sense of the value of a return to the relative concreteness of vital impulses, let us now turn to brief clinical vignettes that show some instances of palpable historical beginnings of human subjects where

there is some semblance of *premature closure*. To that end, let us deploy
the sense of emotional and physical *dislocation* in our subjects as metaphor for historical accounts where premature interpretation forecloses the
powerful evocativeness of meaning that is faithful to the mind of an Other.
Let us use three clinical vignettes to feed our imagination as we observe
instances of dislocation prematurely interpreted, syntheses made too soon,
as Bachelard would say.

First, an adult patient who revisits a memory of seeing her mother's
dead body dragged out of a river when she was three. It is the story of her
mother's suicide. She comes to treatment with a theory that her mother
was too selfish to care about her and to raise her. The young psychiatrist,
my supervisee, follows the patient's mind in addressing the patient's sense
of abandonment by an allegedly "selfish" mother. Soon, a family story
emerges from an aunt that says that "actually, the mother may have been
killed." Subsequently, the patient's original theory of a "selfish" mother
evolves into this: "If she were murdered, then, maybe, I can forgive her."
Then, she fluctuates between her indictment of her mother as a selfish
person who abandons her little girl and the impossibility of forgiving her
mother. I ask the psychiatrist to pause and to explore with the patient, at
the next opportunity, what *the sense of dislocation in se, as remembered,*
was *for her*. It was not until the clinician could explore the fidelity of the
patient's own experience that treatment could advance. For the first time
she could bring into the treatment family stories of her *refusal to walk* and
her persistent tendencies of *biting everything in sight*, in protest, and *in a
return to vital impulses*, as it were.

Here is a second example of a return to beginnings before treatment
could begin in earnest. We are in the late 70s. I am a student at the Anna
Freud Centre, London, studying to become a child and adolescent psychoanalyst. At a diagnostic conference, an eight-year-old child is being
assessed with a view to the treatment of his encopresis, invariably soiling before he could get to the toilet. An impressive clinical team of faculty, students, and guests who are psychoanalysts, mostly from the United
Kingdom and the United States, have come together, as was customary
at the Anna Freud Centre. After about an hour of the most sophisticated
accounts of the collective wisdom of various clinicians with their various
theories underlying the patient's encopresis, Anna Freud wisely and independently asks: "Has anyone noticed that *this eight-year-old child cannot
read?*" The group is stunned by the apparent simplicity and power of her

question about the potential link between toilet training and verbal fluency. Now, ironically, it is the experts that are dislocated. Anna Freud asks for a student who possesses prior training in the field of learning disabilities to consider teaching the child to read in approximately six months. She asks for a supervising analyst who also has a background in reading disorders to assist with the project before we could resume a clinical assessment for analyzability and psychoanalytic treatment.

A year later I had an opportunity to analyze my first case of encopresis that was remarkably similar to the previous case. The only major difference was that my child patient could read. Now let us go to the intrapsychic story of my case of a seven year old boy. When analysis begins, his first drawings are about a pathway that was a dead-end at the destination, and a dead-end upon his return to where he originally started. In time, he could disclose to his analyst that going to school had been *a dislocating* experience because he could not read *to his satisfaction*; returning home was an equally dislocating experience because he was returning home to scenes of turmoil and family dysfunction. Before he could learn to read to his satisfaction, he soiled himself on the way to school as well as on his way back home. After reading competencies were fully established, he soiled on his way back home. Shortly after analysis began, the soiling stopped at both ends. A whole series of drawings of pathways such as that of the digestive tract in his play and representational world became part of his emerging symbolic world. Toward that symbolic end, vehicles he constructed had to have equal weights in the front and in the back. No imbalance that could lead to danger must occur. He soldiered on toward that symbolic end suffused with sublimation potential. Toward the end of treatment, his teacher wrote to the parents in his school report as follows: N

> sees his picture as a whole and the result is therefore quite powerful. He can convey weight, strength, or other *intangibles* in his drawings and painting. . . . He is capable of thought beyond the obvious. His enthusiasm and ideas and drive make him a good leader. His abilities artistically and physically assist him in achieving high personal satisfaction.

N could now become *centered*. He came to see me at age seven and was quite *dislocated*, soiling himself to and from locations of tension and anxiety. At nine, and by his declaration, he had become "the Field Marshall of the anti-girls' club." Now, he is *in full control of his sphincters, in charge of a world of vital impulses, and in full command* of his emerging *symbolic world*.

Now, let us return to a *concrete dislocation in his history*! In such a return, we are not looking for a genetic fallacy of causality but rather a phenomenology that allows us to grasp the intentionality of *his own constituted* presentation of the events of history. When he was four, he was crossing the street with his mother. He said it was *unsafe to cross*. His mother said it was *safe* to do so. He was hit by a car. He soiled himself in terror. A small scar on his forehead now makes sense; a mark that conceals and unconceals a personal story, behold! The continuity between the physically dislocating experiences in his history and the sublimation of his trauma in the course of treatment. Witness the reconfiguration of cars with balanced bumpers and the teacher's independent testimony of his new demonstrations of competencies and articulation of accounts of weight, strength, and other intangibles in his drawings at school.

In a third clinical vignette, E is a nine-year-old girl referred to me to treat her for her *accident-prone* behavior. As reported by her parents, she has been *running into things* ever since she could walk, often receiving serious injuries as a result of *banging her head* into the edge of furniture. At age nine she has not stopped *getting injured*. In the eyes of her parents, it is more than being clumsy. In their own words, *"there is something more."* Treatment did not reveal anything remarkable about her sense of dislocation, *in se*. Rather, much of the treatment was about the value *she* placed on *being with an Other* who paid close attention to her mind, Moi. She enjoyed explaining things to an adult and beamed with smiles when she felt she had taught me something I had not known. She loved to sit close to me while she explored material that intrigued her. Treatment ended after one year when she was restored to where she should developmentally be, a latency age child who could create games and enjoy rules and the *rules* of *a* game, among other developmental indices. *Rules gave her boundaries*, as it were. It is as if she came into treatment to establish rules for herself: treatment as an epistemic place for discovering rules as emerging tools for anchoring herself and establishing new border frontiers of "go" and "no-go areas," as it were.

At age 16, however, her parents brought her back to me for a consultation because *she had failed her driving test twice and was not likely to pass a third time.* This time I referred her to Colonel Leonard, a local army veteran who had a private driving school for teenagers who needed *something extra* to learn to drive. I also could not take her back into treatment because, after her treatment, her father insisted that it was *his* turn to be analyzed by me. *It was his "turn,"* he declared. He refused to see any other analyst. I analyzed him for six and a half years. It was after his analysis that the request for a consultation for the daughter who could not pass her driving test came.

Whereas the meaning of the dislocation was not evident in the treatment of the child, a major and dramatic dislocation was to be found in *her father's* analysis. Her father had killed his brother in an accident when the father was a pubertal adolescent boy. In his mid-40s, he was now ready to come to terms with the consequences, the length and breadth of his trauma that eventually brought him *physically stooping*, literally, into analysis. When he first entered the room in his stooping posture, the Latin for sending a convicted man *under the yoke* (sub iugum mittere) in Roman times came to mind. We shall return later to a brief vignette from the father's treatment. An account of a major dislocation *deferred*; nachträglichkeit, par excellence!

Upon returning to a vignette from the father's treatment, we shall link dislocation of the subject to the reception of the call that precedes an errand. In short, and to get a little ahead of ourselves, my provisional position in this chapter is that *a dislocation* of the subject occurs when a *subject receives a call*; *the call precedes a summons*; the *summons precedes a mandate; an otherwise and increasingly unshakable response defines the posting of the subject; at length, a pluperfect errand shall have already taken place*. Now we may bracket and suspend this link between the call that, unbeknown to the subject, dislocates and the pluperfect errand that returns the subject to oneself. In order to unpack the process of psychical deferral, let us use the following operational format.

Let us initially visit the work of Martin Heidegger, the German existential phenomenologist and a former student of Edmund Husserl, the founding father of the modern philosophical discipline of phenomenology, in order to get a deeper sense of the *thrownness of the dislocated subject*. The French phenomenologist Jean Luc Marion follows to provide a view of *the subject that is decentered by saturated phenomena* and yet *held at the center*. Finally, a hermeneutic phenomenologist, Claude Romano, follows Marion to demonstrate that *the subject can reconfigure one's world*.

The point here is that Heidegger's account of *thrownness* by itself is insufficient, Marion's subject is too deeply *ensconced in saturation*, and Romano's is a necessary predicate to Heidegger's and Marion's accounts of the experience of the subject.

My project, then, is to touch Heidegger, Marion, and Romano without fully engaging them in the expatiation of my account of the pluperfect errand as a clinical concept that dwells in the epistemic gap between phenomenology and psychoanalysis. It is this triadic sequence of (1) *thrownness* into indebtedness, as in Heidegger; (2) an awakening from a sense of a *decentered saturation* of the subject, as in Marion; and (3) a *reconfiguring*, as in Romano, by the subject as *an act of emancipation* that subserves my clinical project. If we could apprehend the fate of the subject through narratives of thrownness as described by Heidegger, narratives of dislocation from saturation as articulated by Marion, and narratives of reconfiguration as in Romano, we may loosen the grip of the *unwelcome guest turned host* in order to avert *the demise of the subject into* a ghost, a revenant, a subject that disappears and a figure that returns.

Now let us explore three forms of dis-location [sic] in (1) a subject that is thrown and *dislocated by a call* as in Heidegger, (2) forms of *dislocation by saturation* in Marion, and (3) vicissitudes of configuring and reconfiguring the eventness of *dislocation in the form of dispossession* as in Romano. We must do so in order to discover the engine that begins the dislocation: *the call, a call that inaugurates a transgenerational pro-ject, a command deferred, a mandate that will reappear in the thick of a transference in a different form and in a different place.*

A. The "Call of Conscience" to a *Thrown* Entity in Heidegger's *Being and Time*

In Heidegger's analysis, he takes conscience as "*something* which we *have in advance theoretically*," and he considers the formulation of "fundamental ontology" his aim (1962, p. 313). Hence, he will come to treat the appearance of phenomena as *pro-jections* [sic] of the subject. In order to treat conscience as something which we theoretically have in advance and which we must deploy with fundamental ontology in mind, Heidegger will take a few steps to accomplish this aim.

In his own words, "[W]e shall first trace conscience back to its existential foundations and structures and make it visible as a phenomenon of Dasein, holding fast to what we arrived at as that entity's state of Being." Such an ontological analysis is, for Heidegger, "*prior to* any account of *experiences of conscience*" (p. 313; emphasis added.) Notice that such a reduction (Latin, re-ductio, I lead back to) is neither *constituted* as in Husserl's phenomenology nor *leads back to* the *appearance of the phenomena themselves* as in Marion's phenomenology. In such a reduction whose aim is to arrive at an entity's state of being, Heidegger writes, "we must neither exaggerate its outcome nor make perverse claims about it and lessen its worth" (p. 313). Why? Conscience discloses and its disclosure gives us something to understand. *Conscience, as discourse*, then, *reveals itself as a call.* "*That which, by calling . . . gives us to understand is the conscience*" (p. 316).

This call has the character of an *appeal* to Being [sic] *to do something*. The appeal takes the form of *summoning* an entity to "its ownmost Being-guilty" (p. 314). To the *call* of conscience, there must be an entity that does the *hearing*. Our understanding of *the appeal that is heard* shows itself as our *wanting*, as in *lacking*, and as *our desire to have* a conscience, a phenomenon within which lies "the choosing to choose our Being-one's-Self which, in accordance with its existential structure, we call '*resoluteness*'" (p. 314; emphasis in original).

Whence cometh this call of conscience? Penetratingly and decisively, the "call comes *from* me and yet from *beyond me and over me*" (p. 320; italics in original). How may we understand that which comes from me and from *beyond me* and *over me*? Heidegger answers as follows: "Only the existential constitution of *this* entity can afford us a clue for interpreting this kind of Being of the 'it' which does the calling" (p. 320; italics in original).

Cryptically, Heidegger defines the caller as follows:

> The caller is Dasein in its uncanniness: primordial, thrown Being-in-the-world as the "not at home"—'that-it-is' in the "nothing" of the world. The caller is unfamiliar to the everyday they-self. It is something like an *alien* voice.
>
> (p. 322; emphasis in original)

Essentially, an individualized Self is thrown into an unfamiliar nothing; brought into its *there*, "*not of its own accord*" (p. 329; emphasis added).

The idea of *choosing to choose* in Heidegger's existential structure gives the entity considerable agency. Being *thrown into an alien place* renders the entity *without anchor*. The call to conscience that somewhat promised that we may discover the caller as an entity that comes from me, and from beyond me and over me comes to an aporia as a promise left unfulfilled. My search for a *link between the call and an errand* remains unfulfilled. Why is my search unfulfilled?

Heidegger's idea that something comes from me, something comes from beyond me and over me remains *centered in my self-same intrinsic world*. I am looking for an archaic entity that comes before and begins the process of psychical transfer. Parenthetically, in Husserl's phenomenology, we would paraphrase his constitutive project as follows: "how does a subject transform the *events* of history into a *sense* of history?" Where is *the beginning*? Where is *the command* that begins the process of psychical transfer and at length becomes one's own in Heidegger?

For now, we may baldly sum up Heidegger's thesis as follows. Conscience may feel like an alien voice talking to me, and it is not. Rather, it is a silent call that brings me back to myself. What subserves this uncanny call of conscience? The call bespeaks our thrownness into the world, a pro-jection with a Heideggerian dash, as it were, that makes us want, lack, and therefore be indebted, thrown into a surfeit of pangs of compunction, fraught with guilt, and subsequently answerable to a sense of responsibility. In understanding the call, then, humans choose to have a conscience. To be human is decidedly to understand the call of conscience, to want to have this responsibility, and, consequently, become resolute.

Two contemporary French thinkers depart from Heidegger. Jean Luc Marion and Claude Romano appropriate the thrownness of the subject but distinctively depart from Heidegger in their account of the vicissitudes of the projection. A subject can be thrown in Heidegger, but its situatedness, its *location*, its experience of active and passive, the fate of its intentionality, and destiny are decisively different in Marion and Romano.

Marion expatiates his phenomenology of the subject's experience of the phenomenal world in *Reduction and Givenness: Investigations of Husserl, Heidegger and Phenomenology* (1989/1998), *In Excess: Studies of Saturated Phenomena* (2001/2002), and *Being Given: Toward a Phenomenology of Givenness* (1997/2002). Romano turns to a hermeneutic phenomenology to address the vicissitudes of the human subject in *Event and*

World (1998/2009), *Event and Time* (199/2012), and *There Is: The Event and the Finitude of Appearing* (2003/2016).

Marion (2002) sees the subject as *decentered*. But, contra Heidegger, the destabilized subject *is held* at the center, "placed where what gives itself shows itself, and there, it discovers itself given to, and as a pole of givenness, where all the givens come forward incessantly" (Marion, 2002, p. 322). Marion will put forward his idea of saturated phenomena which decenter the subject, invert intentionality, and thus impact the categories of active and passive.

B. The Structure of Experience of the Subject in Marion. Or, the Subject Is Decentered *and* Held at the Center

If saturated phenomena and their *inversion of intentionality* impact the categories of active and passive, how and why does this happening occur?

The *subject* that experiences saturated phenomena receives and endures a call. Due to that call, "*some gift happens to me* because *it precedes me* originarily in such a way that I must recognize that *I proceed from it*" (p. 270; emphasis added). The subject receives and endures the call and its claim as *already given*. For Marion, then, "to speak always and first amounts to passively hearing a word coming from the Other" (p. 270).

Marion takes us to the domain of the *pluperfect* and alters our sense of *activity and passivity* as well as *event and time*. Thus, the call gives me, the call gives me *to myself*, and the call *individuates me*. How? Before encountering and knowing an object in a surprise, before seeing the Other in an interlocution, I am *already* changed into a me under the impact of a call as summons.

Marion comes close to and stops short of using the word "errand" to describe the sequence of responding to a call and returning to oneself. It would be the poet W.H. Auden and his poem "On This Island" that would get me started on this journey of pursuing a greater understanding of the vicissitudes of errands and how they link up to agency and disloca-tion. Inscribing Auden then, we have the following sequence: (1) subject receives a *call*; (2) now the called becomes a *receiver*; (3) the receiver *claims the call*; (4) the call is given as a *summons*; (5) the receiver is *gifted*; (6) the facticity of the *donation* shall have *already* taken place; (vii) sub-ject returns to self; (7) upon the return to oneself after an *errand, subject is changed,* having found oneself in the Other that summoned and sent the subject. Let us make a mental note. Something has changed here from Marion to Auden, from dethronement of the subject to a *bifurcation* of the experience of being decentered *and* being posted on an errand.

A clinical vignette could feed our imagination regarding what a human subject can undergo when saturation is at play. Now let us return to the father of the accident-prone child that came to me for treatment. Let us go back to the pubescent adolescence of this father.

What phenomenon could be more *saturated* than the experience of a pubescent adolescent boy killing his younger brother? What a saturated *event*! This is the memory of the 12-year-old who grew up to explore his history of trauma in a psychoanalysis over which I presided when he was in his 40s. I shall paraphrase such a vignette from the analysis and be as faithful to *his* mind as I can in order to present an episode from his own childhood.

> Once upon a time, *a four-year-old was playing* in a relatively *orderly* way in a sandbox. A two-year-old brother *of his* came to play in that same sandbox in a very *disorderly* way. Grandmother watched with consternation. *She called out his name* as if to say "Isaac! Stop!" She declared that one day when this two-year-old grew up, he would be quite "a terror to deal with." The four-year-old stored his grandmother's *vocative declaration* in his head. He appropriated the declaration as *his own* resolute *call to duty.* He remembered this story in the fourth year of his analysis when he was exploring *his own idea* that his killing of his brother was an act of reciprocity. "*I killed Isaac; he killed me back. From his grave,* he *changed* my life." Hence his own mental paralysis.

In this enigmatic recall, there is a declension of the self, as it were. There is the nominative case of *the subject* who initially played with some order and the accusative case of the disorderly boy that became *the object* of his and grandmother's aggression; the younger child that he killed. There is the performative vocative of a grandmother *calling out* a disorderly child's name to stop creating disorder. There is the genitive relation of his brother as *kin* to himself. There is the dative case of sending his brother *to the grave* to stop him, at grandmother's bidding. There is the ablative case of the murdered child's return *from the grave* (revenant) to kill him back.

Agamben, following Hegel, conceives of "declension as the movement of *the ab-solute; a circle that returns into itself,* the circle that presupposes its beginning and reaches it only at the end" (Agamben, 1999; Hegel, 1977). The self in all its permutations is here in a cryptic memory that descends uneasily into a *declension of roles.*

Behold, grandmother's *script* and a grandson's *appropriation* that comes out of the declension: *the disorderly must die.* In contrast, the *orderly must live, albeit uneasily.* The tension dwells in his adult life as *a sublimation that must not be easily resolved: one must write about love and death that walk hand in hand.* This coexistence opens the door for a potential emancipation from the perceived or received pressure to kill to a representational world that now drives a volition to become freer as a writer to write in tense spaces where *protagonists are both decentered and held at the center.*

C. From the Subject as *Adonné* in Marion to *Advenant* in Romano; or, From a Saturated, Upended Subject to a Configuring Subject That Advances From Presentations of an Event to Represented *Evential* Phenomena

How are events *eventialized* leading to a *structural delay in Romano's work?* Contra Heidegger, an event in Romano's account becomes *evential* [sic] in a *reconfigured* experiential world when something radically changes a subject's external fields of reference into internal fields of reference. *Events as evential then overturn preexisting possibilities* so that we can *reconfigure the world anew.* Subject to no universe of prior possibilities, *an event as evential acquires a new meaning* and *attains a structure* over time and this structure can be interpreted. This interpretation is the *hermeneutic dimension* of Romano's phenomenology.

Consequently, an evential rendition exercises a structural delay in the process of staging historical, cultural, and individual memories from archaic places into the present now. What subtends this structural delay? I notice five considerations that apply in Romano's hermeneutic account of the structural delay.

First, there is the first component of Romano's account of the evential meaning of birth as originary *dispossession*: originary because it pre-dates the birth of the child and its capacity for agency.

For Romano, an advenant is born in the mutation of meaning-making from event to eventual where *I discover myself deprived of settledness*, deprived of interpretive settledness, having been *thrown into a gap* in the "world." Now Romano would claim that *at the core of this adventure, birth radically sets up a gaping fissure that will never again be closed.*

A second component of Romano's account explores further what belies this structural delay when birth is a pre-personal history. *Dispossessed at birth, to be born is nevertheless to be connected to history.* This second component is a paradox: the subject is dispossessed *and still* connected to history. For Romano (2009), then, to be born is on one hand, "*to have a history before having one's own history*: a *prepersonal history*, literally unable to be taken over, introducing into the human adventure an excessive meaning that is incommensurable with my projections and thus radically inexhaustible"(p. 78; italics added). On the other hand, the human subject will always speak of its birth in the orbit of its prepersonal history as follows: "*I was born.*" I will never be able to say that I was the agent of my birth, but I can shape and reconfigure the received. This capacity for each child-subject to shape its own history is why in clinical work we say that three children from the same family who have experienced the same history do not have the same psychological parents.

A third component of what belies a structural delay is the inaugural dissymmetry of *naming.*

Originally dispossessed at birth, born into a prepersonal history, the subject is about to be dispossessed once again. Romano's own words are apt:

> *to be named is to be anticipated by the verbal initiative of another, called by a word that overhangs me and that I cannot completely appropriate, since my name, symbol of my ownership, [symbol] of my "identity," is at the same time, symbol of this initial dispossession.*
>
> (2009, p. 80; emphasis added)

After dispossession, and this is not in Romano, subject is sent on an errand (see Apprey, 1993). The subject that goes on an errand returns to its introjected self. The subject that returns to self, *advenant*, must return to its own creation of *the figure* from whom the mandate came and hence the introjected self. Precisely because one returns not to the sender but to the introjected self, *the categories of active and passive are now overturned.* Romano (2009) coins a word to represent this overturning of active and passive: "passibility" (p. 72).

The fourth and penultimate component of that which belies structural delay, then, is "passibility." What belies this penultimate structural delay? If *passibility* precedes active and passive, what happens to a subject's sense of time? In Romano (2009), then, *passibility* is "being exposed beyond measure to events that cannot be expressed in terms of passivity but *precedes the distinction between active and passive*" (p. 72; emphasis added).

If to be born and named is to be dispossessed; if the subject is sent on an errand; if passibility precedes the categories of active and passive, and if the subject returns to its introjected self, what happens to the subject's sense of time? The pluperfect tense is evoked in Romano's account.

The last component of structural delay inscribes *a pluperfect sense of always coming after* into his schema. If to be born is to be connected to history, and if I am not my own origin, a destiny all too laid out and pre-assigned to me, we are in the realm of *a future anterior.* So, poignantly, for Romano (2009),

> if I cannot take over this past, if this prepersonal past, coming before all memory and forgetting, preceding birth and opening to it, *is a plu-perfect I always "come after*," it is *also what makes possible always "go before" me and thus well up from the future.*
>
> (p. 78; emphasis added)

Accordingly, we have a turbulent and pluperfect errand when, ab initio, sub-ject is posted on an originary mandate. Then, sub-ject undergoes a passibility that precedes active and passive. Next, having accepted an errand, sub-ject becomes a figure into whom ancestral and toxic misrepresentation or an aberrant representation is stored. Subsequently, sub-ject adheres to a peremptory return because it is still on an errand and *has to return.* Finally, when sub-ject does return to itself after a structural delay, we have *a motivated and turbulent pluperfect errand.*

Antecedent and Consequent Dislocations Reconfiguring Originary Figures and Facsimiles of Original Figures Into a *Spiral Circularity*

Following Romano, our birth is the *originary dispossession* of ourselves. Second, we are paradoxically connected *and* disconnected to someone else's history. Third, the moment we are named, we are *possessed and dispossessed*. Fourth, *an originary* [sic] *dispossession* of oneself and *an original* [sic] *possession* of oneself *are juxtaposed in an unstable disequilibrium; a disequilibrium* that accompanies an ecstatic sense of standing outside oneself. Fifth, I am pre-dated in ways where *I cannot take over my past. Now, active and passive alternate.* Henceforth, *I am stuck with a pluperfect sense of always coming after.*

In the clinical relationship, then, a new and public space is created. In this new place, subject creates *new versions of original creations in the transference* where the analyst is made to *stand in* for an anterior figure. As the transference intensifies, the originary project of an anterior figure catches up with the recent and original creation of the subject. Jacques Lacan (1966, 1969, 1971) describes this sequence as follows: Scene I catches up with Scene II in an "après-coup," a phenomenon Freud (1895) originally called "Nachtraglichkeit," which tends to be insufficiently translated into English as deferred action. Lacan's account of après coup to translate "Nachtraglichkeit" bespeaks circular and apparent causality. However, the preponderance of dispossession, disconnection, disequilibrium, alternation of active and passive, interrupts the circularity of departure and return. The subject's life journey with its myriad catalogue of dispossession of self as rupture, followed by a suture to foster a negotiated rupture in anticipation of a return to self-same subject, among other twists and turns, cannot be a circle. A *circle suggests completion* upon return to self when the history of Scene I catches up with Scene II in an "après-coup." Now uneasy departures and returns constitute a *spiral circularity*, where a perennial dislocation mandates *repeated journeys in a never completed series of postings and returns.*

The poet T.S. Eliot (1943) seductively teases us in Four Quartets with an essence in which he declares that what we call the beginning is quite often the end. To constitute an end is paradoxically to create a beginning. The end, then, is where we start from. Accordingly, at the end of our explorations, we come to know that the end is where the journey began, and we get to know that self-same destination for the first time.

In knowing the place for the first time, the circle is broken into a spiral circularity. When we know the place whence we departed for the first time, we can begin to reconfigure and to *resubjectivize* an errand again and again until we shall have acquired a measure of emancipation from historical postings by anterior and appositive subjects. In knowing the place for the first time and in a newly reconfigured way, our *exit strategy* from constructed, constituted, or induced dislocated and toxic errands shall have begun.

In Place of a Conclusion; or, Circling Back to a Delayed Preface

When a subject is decentered and held at the center, following Marion, there is, nevertheless, a dislocation that saturates that entity. When there is a "call of conscience" to that thrown entity, as in Heidegger, there is the dislocation of a call that summons an Other *to do something*. There is, precisely, *an errand.* When the subject is possessed and dispossessed, as in Romano, there is a dislocating upheaval that changes the position of self and other, the sense of time from linear to pluperfect. By the time the subject shall have realized the errand, it is already too late to control its toxicity. Now we need the idea of *reciprocal connection* in Husserl's *Experience and Judgement* (1948) and the clinical experience of *reciprocal correction* to make change possible in the clinical setting. When an archaic call is made to a subject in dream, or in the transference or in a psychologically charged external world event, a clinician can hear the weight of the dislocating errand *with* a subject in a new, public, and shared space.

Thanks to the new and public space in the clinical setting, the entity that listened to the originary call will come to know that perception is communalized in ways where there is a constant *alteration, revision,* and *co-creation of meanings* of the received and perceived phenomenon through *reciprocal connection* and, I wish to emphasize, *reciprocal correction.*

Decentering of the human subject, then, includes a series of dislocations, subsequentiality, and spiral circularity until the subject shall have arrived at some sustainable, sublimated, and tolerable place of closure *in the presence of a new and clinically informed Other who would stay alive for the anguished sub-ject* [sic]. *Staying centered for a dislocated Other, co-creating meanings, empowering the listener to hear differently and at one's own emancipating pace, revising the call and with one's own agency, hearing the call in multiple and in life-sustaining ways, is precisely the aggregate praxis for* loosening the grip of an alien guest turned host that calls for and scripts the demise of a subject.

Staying alive for a dislocated subject, however, does not mean that the analyst as listener is not thrown, from time to time. Rather, in the process of making meaning of the vicissitudes of dislocation, clinician and patient alike can become *fellow seekers*, as it were, as they negotiate processes of reciprocal connection and reciprocal correction. *A symbolic order wherein subject is empowered to resubjectivize the injected toxic errand may now drive the creation of an* **exit strategy** *from an archaic mandate to die or from structures of experience that trap and destroy the self.*

References

Agamben, G. (1999). Se: Hegel's Absolute and Heidegger's Ereignis. In *Potentialities*, pp. 116–137. Palo Alto, CA: Stanford University Press.

Apprey, M. (1993). Dreams of urgent/voluntary errands and transgenerational haunting in transsexualism. In *Intersubjectivity, Projective Identification and Otherness*, eds. M. Apprey & H. Stein. Pittsburgh, PA: Duquesne University Press.

Bachelard, G. (1979). *Lautréamont*. Dallas, TX: The Dallas Institute Publications (Orig. 1939).

Eliot, T. S. (1943). *Four Quartets*. New York, NY: Faber and Faber.

Freud, S. (1895). Project for a scientific psychology. In *Standard Edition*, Volume 1, pp. 281–391. London: Hogarth Press.

Hegel, G. W. F. (1977). *The Phenomenology of Spirit*. Oxford: Oxford University Press, p. 488; Agamben, 1999, p. 118.

Heidegger, M. (1962). *Being and Time*. Translated by J. Maquarrie & E. Robinson. New York: Harper and Rowe.

Husserl, E. (1948/1973). *Experience and Judgment*. Evanston, IL: Northwestern University Press.

Lacan, J. (1966). *Écrits*. Translator by B. Fink. New York: Norton, 2007.

Lacan, J. (1969). *Séminaire XVI, D'un Autre à l'autre*. Paris: Seuil.

Lacan, J. (1971). Discours de conclusion au Congrès de l'École Freudienne de Paris sur "La technique psychanalytique." *Lettres de l'École freudienne*, 1972(9): 507–513.

Marion, J.-L. (2002). *Being Given: Toward a Phenomenology of Givenness*. Palo Alto: Stanford University Press.

Romano, C. (2009). *Event and World*. New York: Fordham University Press.

Chapter 11

"Containing the Uncontainable"

The Return of the Phantom and Its Reconfiguration in Ethnonational Conflict Resolution[1]

A phenomenologically informed psychoanalytic praxis for framing and conducting ethno-national conflict resolution in fractured communities or disturbed organizations is presented. In this chapter, the context is limited to a broader ethnonational conflict resolution within one country but with the shadow of an empire that once ruled this self-same nation.

When conducted with care, it begins with the polarization of each side in the conflict and continues into a second phase where the antagonism changes into the negotiation of paradox, irony, and multiplicity of positions. Third, the crossing of mental borders with trepidation follows. Finally, an ethic of responsibility, where common ground is sought brings closure to the process. A plea for humility, however, is required of practitioner scholars of conflict resolution because there are invariably phantoms of history that threaten to return to derail what at one time looked like success long after the work shall have been formally completed. *The return of ancestral grievances requires practitioners to seriously consider implications for follow-up.*

Operational Format of the Chapter

This chapter proposes that there will always be conflict in ethnonational relations, but *we have to have structured psychopolitical processes in place to ensure that conflict does not become maladaptive or malignant.*

Historical grievances that are sedimented are embedded in contemporary politics as though an archive exists to conceal both past and present unconscious mental content. These sedimentations are reactivated into modern contexts. Subsequently, they are extended to do the higher bidding of serving new and contemporary purposes. To ensure that conflict does not become malignant, psychopolitical dialogue must shift antagonistic

DOI: 10.4324/9781003389026-12

politics into agonistic, metaphorical and even playful and plural ways of conceiving and reconfiguring conflict. In the process, *absolute* forms of conceiving alterity or otherness must shift into *relative* alterity. To that end the specific movement must encompass the following four steps: (1) antagonistic polarization between the feuding factions to serve both defensive and adaptive purposes; (2) the discovery that the factions are not homogeneous but heterogeneous parties with paradoxical and even ironic situations, histories, and projects; (3) the crossing of mental borders where the two factions venture to encounter each other with trepidation and retreat from the ventured rapprochement in a back and forth way until they discover agonistic playfulness that opens up new spaces for reconfiguring their conflicts; and (4) the ethic of responsibility that now allows the factions to recognize that they may not agree but can and must, let us say, trade together for their common good. Follow-up of the psychopolitical dialogues must occur in order to ensure that the ghosts of the ancestors, as it were, do not return to wreak havoc in contemporary times with a change of function. The peremptory or paradoxically urgent/voluntary errands behind the spectral return precisely constitute the threat that makes otherwise containable conflict "uncontainable."

I have entitled this chapter "Containing the Uncontainable: The Return of the Phantom and Its Reconfiguration in Ethnonational Conflict Resolution" for three reasons. I want to preserve a healthy tension between what can be realistically expected of human beings who nurture historical injuries and the limits of our capacity as human beings to overturn our received history. Second, I want to substantially extend previous works that now look like outlines of my praxis into a mature praxis that begs for a plea of humility because the power of ancestral voices behind interethnic conflict is a serious omission in earlier writings (Apprey, 1996, 2001).

Third, "Containing the uncontainable" also alerts us to the work of French phenomenologist Jean-Luc Marion (2002), who writes about the subject's saturation and excess of given phenomena. For example, the 1940 Soviet occupation of Estonia is an event, a powerful event with a surfeit of passions that remain to this day. For that reason, Marion asserts that the event of a historical event is experienced by an entire population. Because of the saturation and terror attached to that event, the meaning of an historical event cannot be grasped by a single interpretive gesture. Psychoanalytically, the meaning is overdetermined. Phenomenologically, a defining event such as an occupation imposes itself on the collective memory of an occupied people, current or former, in a way that exceeds any singular aspectual intentional directedness and fills their horizon with multiple expectations. In Marion's words: "The plurality of horizons practically forbids constituting the historical event into one object and demands substituting an endless hermeneutic in time, the narration is doubled by a narration of narratives" (2002, p. 229).

In the field of conflict resolution, if events are saturated and fill the subjects with saturation of passions and terror, the facilitator can also be filled with a surfeit of emotions. For that reason, The facilitator who writes about one's work has to give an account of one's phenomenological presence at both the *experiential* and *conceptual* levels before bracketing, suspending, and deferring one's own phenomenal world in order to begin the process of dispassionately unpacking, without presupposition, the saturation in the process of conflict resolution. Here, then, are my *experiential* and *conceptual* basic assumptions that threaten to inject themselves into the investigation: one driven by my patients' responses to 9/11 and my own response to theirs, the other of a conceptual nature. These would subsequently be bracketed so that we could resume the account of the conflict resolution intervention steps and the plea for humility when historical phantoms return to potentially derail our work after intervention.

Experiential Phenomenological Presence

To the rubrics of "growth and turbulence in the container-contained relation" and "containment, terror and transformation in the large group context," I bring an experiential phenomenological presence. That phenomenological presence can best begin with a powerful anecdote. On the morning of September 11th, a patient walked in for his analytic session. Instead of going straight to the couch as was his usual custom, he paused in the middle of the room, stood still, and as though he were paralyzed, sank into the sofa nearest to him. He spoke as follows: "I don't think I can lie down on the couch today." He sat still, and a few moments later, I replied somberly: "What is new about what humans are capable of doing to one another?" A few more moments later he stood up, having shaken off the paralysis, as it were, and proceeded to the couch with recalcitrant resignation.

From the couch came the following, as though I had given him implicit permission to speak his mind about what human beings are capable of doing to one another: "Actually I am glad the rascals from Wall Street who live in Scarsdale, NY, got killed. My sister-in-law and her husband live in Scarsdale and her husband works on Wall Street." I do not wish to go into the patient's intrapsychic story but to reflect briefly on my own response— "What is new about what humans are capable of doing to one another?"

My response came from an epistemic site of tension between an informed skepticism and an equally resilient belief that humans are capable of transforming the received. This is a tension I do not wish to resolve, but I do wish to hold both sides in an agonistic situation of conflict. I shall elaborate on the agon shortly.

I shall now organize my contribution around three parts: (1) the conceptual basic assumptions behind my pre-text, (2) the context of my work in interethnic conflict resolution to demonstrate a framework that effects transformation by ensuring that the conflict in question does not become malignant; and (3) the provisional conclusion where I suggest why interethnic conflict may be saturated by the phantoms of history. Be that as it may, *the thread that runs through my contribution is the organizing ethical position that there will always be conflict in ethno-national relations but one must ensure that the conflict does not become malignant by creating structures for the resolution of the conflict.*

Pretext: Conceptual Phenomenological Presence

In a somewhat de facto fashion, *terrorists are archivists*, as it were. *They have a very long memory*. Rightly or wrongly, *they try to hold us hostage to their communal memory*, that collective phenomenal world behind their historical grievances. In this sense, as the poet Wallace Stevens would put it, we live in the description of a place but not in the place itself (my paraphrase). In other words, when the grievance is remembered, it would be reanimated with a particular embroidery and a distinct and directed intentionality.

Accordingly, the eminent historian Bernard Lewis alludes to Osama Bin Laden's grievance as one that is framed by his description of three historical events that point to *his sense of* the impotence of the Islamic world in the face of European and Euro American impact. Lewis (2002) writes:

> The impotence of the Islamic world confronted with Europe was brought home in dramatic form in 1798, when a French expeditionary

force commanded by a young general called Napoleon Bonaparte invaded, occupied, and governed Egypt. The lesson was harsh and clear—even a small European force could invade one of the heartlands of the Islamic empire and do so with impunity.

(p. 31)

Egyptians watched helplessly as Napoleon Bonaparte colonized them. Another lesson came a few years later,

> when the French were forced to leave—not by the Egyptians, nor by their Turkish Suzerains, but by a squadron of the Royal Navy commanded by a young admiral called Horatio Nelson. This lesson too was clear; not only could a European power come and act at will, but only another European power could get them out.
>
> (p. 31)

To these two humiliating events Bin Laden would add his discontent about the Israeli occupation of Palestinian land and, for a time, American troops on Saudi soil.

Let us now go to psychoanalysis for another reading of humans as archaic archivists. Two passages speak to this from the work of Heinz Hartmann (1958).

First, humans do not come to terms with their environment anew in every generation. Rather, their relation to the environment is guaranteed by an evolution peculiar to humans, namely the influence of tradition on humans and the survival of the works of man. Hence,

> *we take over from others* . . . *a great many of our methods for solving problems.* . . . The works of man objectify the methods he has discovered for solving problems and thereby become factors of continuity, so that *man lives,* so to speak, *in past generations as well as his own.*
>
> (p. 30; emphasis added)

Hartmann continues with his description of transformation by elaborating on the concept of "change of function" when he suggests that what defensive operations "were once anchored in instincts may subsequently be performed in the service of and by means of the ego, though naturally, new regulations too will arise in the course of the development of the ego and the id" (p. 49) Accordingly, "differentiation progresses not only by creation of new apparatuses to master new demands and new tasks, but also and mainly by new apparatuses taking over, on a higher level, functions which were performed by more primitive means" (p. 50).

Quite baldly, the motor remains the same, but the license plate changes.

Within this horizon of change of function and transformations of acquired history, the French philosopher Maurice Merleau-Ponty (2002) had this to say

> Each [person] has an "*acquired history*" on the basis of the respective ego which is made at home in it. If I am born a sailor's child, then a part of my development has taken place on the ship. But the ship would not be characterized as a ship for me in relation to the earth . . . the ship would itself be my "earth," my homeland. But my parents are not then primordially at home on the ship; they still have the old home, another primordial homeland.
>
> (p. 126; emphasis added)

All this is to say that *there are sedimentations of history* that cry out to be heard. These sedimentations become reactivated in given contexts. The reactivation is subsequently driven by intentionality and extended to serve new and contemporary purposes. (See Apprey, 2006.)

This tier of intentionality can be extended into the political domain and here I will build on the work of the Belgian political scientist Chantal Mouffé, in particular her work "On the Political" (2005).

By the "*political*," Mouffé refers to the dimension of *antagonism* that is inherent in human relations: antagonism that takes many forms and emerges in different types of social relations. For Mouffé, politics constitutes an aggregate of practices, institutions, and discourses that aim to establish a particular order and to organize human existence. It does so in conditions that are invariably potentially conflictual. She considers that when we acknowledge the antagonistic dimension of the political and understand that politics domesticates hostility and tries to defuse antagonism, we can arrive at the central question for democratic politics, the politics of *agonistic pluralism*.

Agonistic pluralism, inter alia, does not eradicate passions in order to promote a rational public consensus; rather, agonistic pluralism tries to tame the passions in order to mobilize contentious debate to serve democratic goals through collective forms of discourse in civil society. *Agonistic pluralism*, then, *searches for alternatives to the existing hegemonic order while it domesticates passions* and, I might add, terror.

Let us now bracket or suspend our phenomenological presence and conceptual basic assumptions in order to provide a context for examining the containment and potential transformation of passion and terror in a large group setting.

The Context of the Conflict Resolution Process in Post-Soviet Estonia

The Center for the Study of Mind and Human Interaction (CSMHI) of the University of Virginia School of Medicine, under the directorship of the psychoanalyst Vamık Volkan was an interdisciplinary center whose work in conflict resolution required the collaboration of psychoanalysts, historians, diplomats, and other scholars. For over two decades, CSMHI was invited to participate in the resolution of conflicts between representatives of nations in conflict. Following the breakup of the Soviet Union, Estonia wished to restore its political independence as well as its psychological independence. CSMHI had participated in other cases with participants from both Russia and Estonia and accordingly became an excellent credible candidate to assist both sides in the process of Estonia's psychopolitical independence from and co-existence with Russia as its neighbor. One account of the methodology for understanding ethnonationalist rituals has been described elsewhere by Volkan (1992). Other accounts of the praxis for presiding over group processes in ethnonational conflict resolution (see Apprey, 1996, 2001) posit four heuristic steps in the conflict resolution process which are meant to be suggestive but not exhaustive or cast in stone. Here, *I will revisit those heuristic steps in order to show the progression from antagonistic to agonistic conflict and potential transformation.* First let us follow the steps that operate in the conduct of ethnonational conflict resolution:

1   Intensive *confidential interviews* are conducted with a cross-section of leaders from all constituencies to ensure that the third-party interdisciplinary interventionists who seek to foster conflict resolution

between the fractured communities understand the historical and contemporary concerns facing Indigenous Estonians and those Russians who have chosen to live in Estonia after the collapse of the Soviet Union.

2   A series of psychopolitical dialogues between representatives of interested parties (20–30 in large, plenary sessions, to open and close each day of talks, and 8–15 people in small work-group sessions) during which lines of communication are opened; concerns are shared; and hidden psychological barriers that separate interested parties are brought to the surface, discussed, and ultimately transformed so that they no longer impede negotiation and movement toward common goals. The process often involves recognizing the influence of historical relationships and events, how they recur, and how they change function when they are perpetuated under different guises to serve new and contemporary purposes. The heuristic steps outlined in this chapter constitute an elaboration of the engagement through psychopolitical dialogue. This second step is essential to the success of step three.

3   In Step 3 the hitherto fractured communities cooperate in the development of, or investment in, specific strategies and projects based on new understanding of the divisive issues that have surfaced during the dialogues. Projects emerge from psychopolitical dialogue based on newly established coalitions between members, the shared needs, and the sense that the implementation of these projects is going to be part of a longer-term process of change. In this third step, projects are undertaken jointly by the parties in conflict, and they do so with input from the third-party facilitators.

4   The third party (CSMHI) withdraws as the community continues working toward common goals through dialogues that complement and support ongoing projects. Now the two groups can form a non-governmental organization (NGO) to institutionalize their ownership of the conflict resolution process. As an NGO, they can raise funds to foster capacity building and sustainability of their joint work. Thus, the fourth step involves projects independently undertaken by the groups hitherto in conflict but without input from the third-party facilitators.

These four parts constitute *the lager methodology of interethnic conflict resolution*. Within that larger frame lie the four heuristic steps that occur in the *small group sessions* of the psychopolitical dialogue (that is, part 2 of the methodology). I shall expatiate on them in the following using the philosopher Mark Taylor as one conceptual mouthpiece.

Some Basic Assumptions Behind the Technical Praxis of Ethnonational Conflict Resolution

Taylor (1987) writes in his introduction to *Altarity* [sic] that "*the history of society and culture is, in large measure, a history of the struggle with the endlessly complex problems of difference and otherness*" (p. xxi, emphasis added). Noting further that this century has been dominated by communism and racism, among other "isms," he treats the issue of difference as decisively political although it is also of psychological, artistic, philosophical, and theological importance. This search for radical otherness and irreducible difference, he insists, obsesses and possesses many of today's most successful thinkers.

Along with Taylor's view, I take the position that in the field of conflict resolution, any conception of the other as fixed or absolute dangerously lends itself to the readiness to dehumanize the other. Nor is the facile notion that "we are one blood" a helpful solution because it poses a threat to a much-needed sense of self stability and differentiation. Of even greater threat to participants in conflict is any notion of self as changing or relative because a precipitous readiness to change poses a threat to a group's identity as well. *The dimension of alterity as process and trajectory between absolute alterity, at the front end of the conflict resolution process, and relative alterity, at the other end, is the current that subserves and runs through this chapter.* Here the dimension of alterity as process of engagement between Self and Other that can potentially make continuity out of the antinomies of absolute and relative alterity will be shown to reveal itself in the arena of conflict enactment and resolution between two feuding factions. I hold the view that *Self as agency is an approximation, the Other as absolute a misnomer, and that when Self and Other engage in a process of resolution of conflict, an ambiguous play space opens up fostering an exchange of representations of Self and Other.*

The Four Heuristic Steps as Waystations of the Trajectory From Absolute to Relative Alterity or From Antagonistic Pluralization to Agonistic Pluralism: Brief Comments About the Small Group Work in the Conflict Resolution Process in Estonia

Four waystations typically occupy that epistemic play space of description and conversation between absolute alterity and relative alterity. The case of Estonia's restoration of independence from Russia amplifies the steps in the trajectory that reveal themselves in the conflict resolution process where two parties are involved in a feud.

What group process emerges when native Estonians and Russian speaking residents backed by Russians from the Russian Federation come together to resolve their interethnic conflicts? After seven four-day meetings over a period of three years, from 1994–1997, the following phases in the evolution of the group process can retrospectively be identified. A previous paper (Apprey, 2001) provides a more comprehensive account of the process. Here a summary is provided only to frame the extension of that previous work.

Accordingly, the group work typically begins with *antagonistic polarization* as a first step.

Phase I: Antagonistic Polarization of Factional Positions: Demonization of the Other

Under the category of polarization, the Other is demonized. The Other is imagined to be a terrible other. That Other has a marginal status. Preconstructed as dangerous, the other is posited in close juxtaposition to the subject's own relatively favored position.

Accordingly, Russians are those who suffer under the hegemony and control of Estonians. They suffer when Estonians inflict alleged "human rights violations" on them. This is the Russian position.

On the Estonian side, the Russian Federation is an obstacle to the fulfillment of Estonian aspirations towards integration into Europe, in particular into NATO. The Russians in contrast are "Asians," "not European" and therefore "not like us" Indigenous Estonians.

Phase II: Differentiation Within Each Faction; or, Suspending Absolute Alterity: Multiplicity of Positions Within Each Faction

Under the rubric of differentiation within each integral faction or self-same subject system, a second phase follows when facilitators have permitted the process of polarization to take place and have allowed it to assume the necessary function of self-definition and clarification of borders between the two sides. Here, differentiation within each side becomes possible because of *the emerging recognition of paradoxes within the self-same subject system's ideological positions.* Here, as De Certeau (1984), Dollimore (1991), and Uebel (2005) indicate, *the border between participants of each faction are recognized as having a double status of marker of separation and a line of commonality within each side.* In this respect *"to be against (opposed to) is also to be against (close up, in proximity to) or, in other words, up against"* (Dollimore, 1991, p. 229, emphasis added). For example, when Estonians fight for Soviets against Nazis who also have Estonians fighting for them, Estonians are against each other, or opposed to each other. Yet, because both sides include Estonians, Estonians are close to each other or, at least, proximal to each other. In short, they are both close to and up against each other.

Phase III: The Threshold of Border Crossing: A Depressive or Manic Shift Toward Relative Alterity

In this third waystation of the two sides negotiating and subsequently crossing mental borders, both sides together encounter the trauma and obsession of their historical grievances. Here, the place or function of dialogue as that which creates mental spaces and, more precisely, opens up new and illusionistic play spaces, presents itself. Borderlines open up and become recognized as potential spaces between two feuding factions. Those gaps or middle spaces, which have now become *illusionistic spaces for bridge building* (Pruyser, 1983), now symbolize exchange and encounter that facilitate an eventual crossing of mental borders. This crossing of mental borders effects the transformation of the trauma and obsession of historical grievances. The third way station is preeminently a place of agonistic playfulness and fantastic metaphorization of conflicting positions admixed with serious dialogue. This crossing of mental borders that transforms trauma and obsession of historical grievances operates in ways where the two sides that had hitherto been polarized now operate conjunctly, and these two sides dialogue in ways where the terms of a binary are correspondent. Here, one term proposes the other for its meaning. The hitherto absolutely Other is integrated to the selfsame subject system through encounter with and resolution of ambivalence. In making complementarities out of antinomies, absence or exclusion simultaneously becomes a presence. It is not until this waystation reaches a peak of metaphorization, with both sides contributing to the new imagery and imagining, that the establishment of common ground can be trusted. When experience in this phase is depressive, there are painful silences accompanied by attempts to cross over the fence, as it were. An evocative description out of this depressive episode was once described by a participant as "a place where a policeman is born." In psychoanalytic terms, a superego is established that enables both sides to operate with a new aim and direction. When there is a manic shift, the two sides crack mythical and folklorist jokes about the other. They laugh hilariously together in recognition of their common humanity.

Phase IV: The Establishment of Ethical and Pragmatic Solutions

In this final waystation of the creation of new and adaptive solutions, *ethical positions of trial actions of mutual responsibility* emerge. These ethical positions lead to pragmatic projects that point to indices of internalization of new and generalizable adaptive solutions.

Accordingly, toward the end of our four-day meetings, the different sides made multiple suggestions about what could be done to mitigate tensions between Russians and Estonians. Some suggestions were realistic, others unrealistic. However, the most common and repeated suggestion was to let the dialogue continue to occur between the different groups of representatives. One step that was intended to break the vicious cycle of inflammatory remarks from Russia and Estonia had already been taken in the course of our work. Between the penultimate session of the third day and the morning of the fourth and last day, the Estonian psychologist had already e-mailed for publication a response to his fellow Estonian, the nationalist Member of Parliament whose newspaper article had inflamed passions in Russia and embarrassed Estonians. The tone and current of the MP's article was destructively aggressive and needed to be tamed and transformed. In Chantal Mouffé's terms, passions needed to be domesticated. The e-mail was intended to balance the MP's views.

Returning to the Dynamic(s) Behind the Four Heuristic Steps That Occur in the Small Group Psychopolitical Process

It was indicated early in this chapter that four typical steps present themselves in the evolution of the conflict resolution in small groups. It was indicated further that these steps turn around the issue of vicissitudes of alterity. Let us now identify the dynamic that links the steps with the vicissitudes of alterity, from absolute to relative Alterity, and to the exchange of Self and Other representations that shows itself in the agonistic metaphorization which in turn permits a credible consensus building process to follow.

Starting with antagonistic polarization where one group demonizes the other in implicit and/or explicit ways, it is essential for the facilitator to recognize that the exorcism of the Other is a first and necessary step. It is necessary for the distinct purpose of defining each group's identity and for situating oneself with a clearer sense of who the subject is; one may know for the moment who the enemy is, or at least who the enemy is thought to be. If this part of the process is accepted as adaptive to begin with, the participants are then able to reveal the anxiety that accompanies each polarized position. In a word, by accepting the initial wall that is built around each faction, each feuding party may then borrow strength from the facilitator(s) to examine how anxiously the wall gets built and maintained. The initial dynamic of demonization of the Other ironically needs to emerge only to be discarded to facilitate entry into the next and second phase in the evolution of the group.

Next, when differentiation within each polar faction emerges, the most helpful dynamic that permits the group to evolve is that of paradox and irony. For example, when Estonians recognize that they were forced to fight on both sides of World War II, a new level of thoughtful reflection replaces the need to demonize the Other. Likewise, Russians come to recognize their heterogeneity. In the process they remind the group that some Russian-speaking Estonians, such as Russian Jews and Old Believers, came to Estonia to flee from Soviet oppression. Others, however, were KGB agents and retired former military officers of the Soviet era. Paradoxes begin to create a new level of empathic reflection within each polar faction as well as across the psychological ramparts each side had created earlier.

In the third step of crossing mental borders, the dynamic of metaphorization in the dialogue between the feuding parties opens up new spaces where new ideas can be played with. Playing and bridge building as illusionistic and *agonistic* processes promote new representations of feuding and consensus building. The inadequation, that is, a sustained and embedded structure of experience that affectively and inadequately describes Russians as wild, non-European Asians who might eat up the enemy, gives way to joining with them to seek mutually beneficial solutions. Conversely, the inadequation of seeing Estonians as vengeful human rights abusers gives way to the recognition of the Other as needing to include Russians in the building of a greater civic society and a democratic country. Of course, the sources of the original conflicts remain, because history cannot be changed, but the participants have the courage to encounter their conflicts and attempt to resolve them. The result of the metaphor-driven and meaningful dialogue that emerges is that there is now a replacement of concrete passions by a new order of designations to which all parties can relate. All parties can relate to the policeman called responsibility, family feud, marital discord, divorce, step-parenting, and so on and so forth. Accordingly, humor and thought can converge to promote a higher level of engaging each other in a situation of conflict as they seek building blocks for consensus building. This is the journey toward a condition that Vamık Volkan (1992) has aptly termed "a vaccination," where they recognize their conflicts and are able to engage each other, but the conflict is no longer malignant. In the fourth phase, they are emotionally free to make ethical statements and join forces to create mutually beneficial projects.

Text: In Place of a Conclusion: The Return of the Phantom to Make the Container "Uncontainable"

Containing the terror and passion subserving ethnonational conflicts is a formidable task. The archival nature of historical grievances causes feuding parties to oscillate between *fading and recall* of their sedimented traumatic histories. These sedimentations of history may be recalled at particularly fractious times when collective memory is charged to be the carrier of historical grievances. That which is reactivated may then be used by leaders or terrorists to serve new and contemporary purposes.

When psychoanalysts, diplomats, and historians, among others, come together to repair fractured communities, the ethic of remembering can be interrogated in a relatively contained setting. In the four-step heuristic praxis described here, practitioners have an opportunity to contain and transform antagonistic politics into an agonistic pluralism that can accommodate the reality that there will always be conflict but mechanisms must be in place to contain the conflict and to arrive at provisional solutions or, at least, a provisional containment of the passions.

So, we have our four-step heuristic model for containing terror and passion in interethnic conflict. I am a witness of its containing value. Estonia's relationship with its Estonian Russians improved. They joined NATO. Their gross domestic product hit #4 in the world at one point. They prospered economically, politically, and psychologically.

But, lo and behold, *phantoms returned from the dead to haunt them*. Some 15 years after the interethnic conflict resolution between the Indigenous Estonians and their Estonian Russians, Estonia had to decide what to do with Russian historical statues and other spectral figures in the hallowed spaces of Estonia. Old tensions were renewed. Manifestly, a Russian statue on Estonian soil represents colonial oppression and transgressions. For Russians, the same statue represents victory over the Nazis. We are back to the archive where historical grievances are deeply sedimented but can be reactivated and extended to serve new and contemporary nationalistic purposes.

Accordingly, the Estonian experience of the return of the phantoms enables us to rethink what an archive is. *Think of the archive as an irrepressible transgenerational memory that, like Janus, simultaneously points to the past and to the future*. In his book *Archive Fever*, Derrida (1995) would maintain the same *tension at the onset* of his argument but later tilt his account of the *archive toward the future*. He writes: "*In an enigmatic sense . . . the question of the archive is not, we repeat, a question of the past*" (p. 36, emphasis added). Rather,

> it is a question of the future itself, the question of a response, of a promise and of a responsibility for tomorrow. . . . A spectral messianicity

is at work in the concept of the archive and ties it, like religion, like history, like science itself, to a very similar experience of the promise.
(p. 36; emphasis added)

Whereas Derrida wants to resolve the tension between the archive as a return to the beginning and the archive as a commanding commencement, I want to keep the tension unresolved. Clinical evidence abundantly shows us that the phantom oscillates between the past unconscious and the present unconscious and thus constantly lures and ambushes us into thinking that we can contain the phantoms in the archive. With a plea of humility, I must maintain that the slippery peremptoriness of the spectral mission makes the attempt to contain the phantom a folly. In short, the formidable presence of the phantom in the past or present unconscious is decisively uncontainable. Accordingly, effort after effort must be made to bring some semblance of order in the "container-contained" reverie without the expectation of enduring peace. There may not be a once-and-for-all resolution. Constant vigilance, follow up, and reconfiguration of projects cry out for new ways to give the phantom a decent burial in its rightful place. This constant vigilance and mutual engagement is a tested way of taking the toxins, as it were, from communal memories that carry toxic or turbulent historical grievances, and thus giving the dead a decent burial, as it were.

Note

1 Apprey, M. (2014). "Containing the uncontainable": The return of the phantom and its reconfiguration in ethnonational conflict resolution. *The American Journal of Psychoanalysis*: 162–175, © 2014, Springer Nature. Reprinted with permission.

References

Apprey, M. (1996). Heuristic steps for negotiating ethnonational conflicts: Vignettes from Estonia. *New Literary History*, 27(2): 199–212.

Apprey, M. (2001). Group process in the resolution of ethnonational conflicts: The case of Estonia. *Group Analysis*, 34: 99–113.

Apprey, M. (2006). Difference and the awakening of wounds in intercultural analysis. *Psychoanalytic Quarterly*, LXXV: 73–93.

De Certeau, M. (1984). *Spatial Stories in the Practice of Everyday Life*. Translated by S. Randall. Berkeley, CA: University of California Press.

Derrida, J. (1995). *Archive Fever: A Freudian Impression*. Baltimore: Johns Hopkins University Press.

Dollimore, J. (1991). *Sexual Dissidence: Augustine to Wilde/Freud to Foucault*. Oxford: Clarendon.

Hartmann, H. (1958). *Ego Psychology and the Problem of Adaptation*. New York: International University Press.

Lewis, B. (2002). *What Went Wrong? Western Impact and Middle Eastern Response*. Oxford: Oxford University Press.

Marion, J.-L. (2002). *Being Given: Toward a Phenomenology of Givenness*. Palo Alto, CA: Stanford University Press.

Merleau-Ponty, M. (2002). *Husserl at the Limits of Phenomenology*. Evanston, IL: Northwestern University Press.

Pruyser, P. (1983). *The Play of the Imagination: Toward a Psychoanalysis of Culture*. New York: International Universities Press.

Taylor, M. C. (1987). *Altarity*. Chicago & London: University of Chicago Press.

Uebel, M. (2005). *Ecstatic Transformations: On the Uses of Alterity in the Middle Ages*. New York: Palgrave Macmillan.

Volkan, V. D. (1992). Ethnonationalistic rituals: An introduction. *Mind and Human Interaction*, 4(1): 3–19.

Chapter 12

"To Maurice, With Best Wishes From One Strategist and Peacemaker to Another. John"

An Evocative Reminiscence of Tension Between a Quiet Psychoanalytic Inner Voice and the Fire Outside

Pretext: Inside and Outside Fold Into Each Other

In this chapter, I want to feed our imagination on what happens outside when the mind is on fire and what happens inside when there is fire outside. To that end, I want to begin with the most evocative metaphor: the fold.

My favorite passage comes from the French scholar Gilles Deleuze. It goes like this:

> The outside is not a fixed limit, but a moving matter animated by peristaltic movements, folds and foldings that together make up an inside: they are not something other than the outside, but precisely the inside of the outside.
>
> (Deleuze, 1986/1988, pp. 96–97)

Representationally, the fold simulates the presentation of thought so that inside space, or, more precisely, internal fields of reference to the outside, are topologically in close contact with outside space so that external fields of reference loop back to the inside. *These two spaces remain in confrontation.* They enter into a constant exchange at that permeable border where inside and outside edge towards each other. This juxtaposition, in turn, causes the fold to become a social event between them. Movement, then, I submit, constitutes an act of going from one fold into another fold in *spiral circularity*.

Context: Passing the Buck to Someone to Wage War

If the fold between internal frames of reference into the external world and, in reverse, the translation of a psychologically charged external world into

DOI: 10.4324/9781003389026-13

a mental world is my pretext, what is the context of this chapter? It is my first face-to-face encounter with the renowned political scientist, John Mearshimer. Why would a psychoanalyst have the occasion to meet a political scientist in the memorable way I am about to describe?

It is the year 2003, and I have taken leave from my teaching responsibilities at the University of Virginia, where I practice as a psychanalyst and teach residents of psychiatry and medical students, in order to study social change management at the Weatherhead School of Management in the Doctor of Management (DM) program. *I am determined to make inside and outside fold into each other in my scholarship as a psychoanalyst and as a practitioner scholar of social change.*

We were fortunate to hear Mearshimer himself speak about his account of why states decidedly compete for power and pursue hegemony (2001). Following his lecture on his brand of realism, I was doubly fortunate to ask him what he thought about nation building and inter-ethnic conflict resolution by third-party negotiators. His answer? "I do not think it is the business of one state to enter into conflict resolution between two states in conflict." Rather, "you must get the indigenous people to do the work themselves." At the end of his talk, and I surmise, realizing how wounded I felt by his answer and given my investment in the field of conflict-resolution, he thoughtfully and empathically autographed his book for me. He wrote, "To Maurice, with best wishes from one strategist and peacemaker to another. John."

Not being a dichotomist, I am constantly looking for ways to build bridges: within political discourse, within psychoanalysis, and between political discourse and psychoanalysis.

So, why would a psychoanalyst seriously wish to engage Mearshimer in the first place?

I was a member of an interdisciplinary group of psychoanalysts, political scientists, diplomats, historians, and others who served as third-party facilitators for Russian and Estonian officials after the Soviet Union fell. We were in Estonia to mediate tensions between Indigenous Estonians and Estonian Russians. In the early stages of the conflict, tensions were palpable. For Russians, too many neighbors of the Russian Federation were already hostile to Russia. Therefore, Russia did not want these former Soviet countries to become members of NATO. They feared a tremendous conflagration would follow. War! It did not happen. After four years of active intervention and two more years of informal follow-up visits, there was no war between Russia and its Baltic neighbors. There have been varying degrees of tension, but no war. Mearshimer, ever the *offensive realist* who would rather have hegemons or their third-party facilitators *pass the buck*, made his position clear. He was wrong *this time*. Our interdisciplinary group of psychoanalysts, political scientists, diplomats, historians, and others facilitated the restoration of independence in Estonia and its membership in the European Union and NATO.

Mearshimer, however, would have his day a decade or so later. Putin took Crimea. Sanctions were imposed. In response to these tensions and anxieties, Mearshimer would still insist that the United States and its allies should abandon their plan to westernize Ukraine and instead aim to make it a neutral buffer.

It is 2022. Putin is invading Ukraine. The world is watching as US and Western European countries practice *offensive realism*: providing weapons for Ukraine to carry out its own fight. As I write this chapter, there are tears in my eyes. I am watching death and devastation. Even if one side wins such a war, it would at best be *a Pyrrhic victory*. In contrast, *Estonia, now a member of NATO, stands relatively secure*, thanks to our interdisciplinary efforts as facilitators and collaborative work with both Indigenous Estonian and Estonian Russian scholars and politicians.

Text: The Privileged Voice of Psychoanalysis

In interdisciplinary work between psychoanalysts and others, there are a number of projects: diagnostic work, large group explorations, small group interventions, and myriad interventions. This part of the chapter is not about our technical work. Rather, *I want to comment on the psychanalytic voice that shielded me from the emotional toll of the work* as I spent four years of travel to Estonia to intervene, and two informal follow-up years.

By psychoanalytic voice, I am referring to such precepts as (1) upending resistance to teaching psychoanalysis to college students, (2) overturning resistance expressed through repression, or (3) hearing psychological pain and choosing when to intervene with an empathic silence or with words. Following are three of the multiple experiences of situations that made me pleased to be a psychoanalyst without necessarily having to practice formal psychoanalysis in a politically hot environment: post-Soviet Estonia.

First Narrative Text: Upending Resistance to Teaching Psychoanalysis

In the third year of the Estonia project, the course director of the Department of Psychology at Tartu University invited me to teach an introductory course on psychoanalysis in one month. As planned, a representative would meet me at the airport and drive me to the university. No one came. I took a two and a half-hour taxi trip to Tartu at my own expense. I took a room at a hotel that Sunday. No one to receive me. On the Monday morning. I went to the department to start teaching. The good news is that at the gate, I recognized the rector of the university. He had visited the University of Virginia in the Soviet days when he was a nationalist. When the USSR fell, he became the rector.

He provided me with the best furnished house for a visiting professor. The bad news is that the course director had changed plans for my one-month introductory course on psychoanalysis. Instead, I was to condense four weeks of teaching into one. This means that I would teach every day for five hours. What else could go wrong? I had bound a volume of psychoanalytic papers that I use for the one-year course I teach to third year post-graduate residents and sent a copy by Federal Express to the department one month ahead of time. Instead of distributing the material to the students as previously planned, she sent the papers to the library. This means that the students could not have read them beforehand. She planned to tell them where to find the papers when I came to class that Monday.

I could have returned to my four-star hotel in Tallinn, done my project, and returned to the United States. Instead, I chose to teach students who had not read one paper on psychoanalysis before then: Freud on Monday, Klein on Tuesday, Kohut on Wednesday, Fairbairn on Thursday, and a summary on Friday.

I transformed my aggression into constructive aggression. As a child analyst, I knew how to protect an analysis from ambivalent parents. I was in a zone. After three hours, one student asked for a break. We resumed and completed Freud, such as I could, in one day. The course was completed with planned breaks, and the work of the whole course got done.

Every evening, I invited the students to a reception in my new house the rector had provided. We had a reception with refreshments, tutorials, and fun conversations. The waitresses were so amazed and pleased, they stood around, ever ready to assist. "No one has ever done this for our students. Thank you!" One evening I went to a shop. An elderly storekeeper stood up and beamed: "You must be the professor from America who is teaching my son. He said he has never sat in a class for three hours without a break."

Four years later I received a letter from a student, saying that at the end of their studies they must write an essay on the best course each student ever took. They were unanimous in their choice: *moi*. Even better, the writer was on her way to London to take her master's degree in psychology with a psychoanalytic orientation.

Second Narrative Text: Let Us Go to That Primal Place Where We Were All Infants Before: Upending Resistance Expressed Through Repression

In the Soviet era, Estonian kindergarten pupils were separated from Russian-speaking kindergartens. In Estonian-speaking kindergartens, there was a quota of one Russian child per four Estonian-speaking children. The manifest reason: Russian children were "boisterous." "They would run all over the quiet Estonians." I discovered in direct observation that they were more alike than different. For example, they all loved playing "Cowboys and Indians."

Our job was to foster integration. They had difficulty coming up with common projects. Before every visit I received information that they had chosen a common project. Upon my return, they had repressed the idea of *that* common project. My plan to break that pattern? Have workshops with them where we all would watch the Robertson films on "Young Children in Brief Separation." The impact on them was profound. They talked openly; they cried together about what they once had, and lost: "In Soviet times if a teacher had a sick child at home, she stayed at home to take care of her child. Now, if she stayed at home she would lose money." After two such workshops, the repression barrier was lifted. They had a project called "Hand-in Hand." The ratio of one Russian child per four Estonians in an Estonian kindergarten changed to three Russian children per six Estonians.

In our work with post-Soviet Estonians and Estonian Russians I was able to hear a psychoanalytic voice that would invariably remind me that I was in the story, but the story was not necessarily about me. I could stay alive for participants in turmoil. I could maintain a psychoanalytic attitude to upend repression resistance to change in a post-Soviet fragile ego.

At the end of the project a lecturer who had been watching the way I worked as a psychoanalyst gave me a gift I could not refuse. The gift was an egg-shaped ornament that one could open and close. Her words: "You have been coming here for four years, sometimes 20 degrees below zero. *You have very delicately listened to us and intervened. When you open an egg delicately, you find a new life.*" The yolk within can serve as symbol of gentle, enduring, and meaningful life, one that has the potential to exceed a Pyrrhic victory or can co-exist, albeit uneasily, with offensive realism.

Third Narrative Text: A Co-Investigator Is in Deep Pain After a Visit to a Mass Gravesite in Klooga, Estonia, for Jewish Ancestors

Two years after the formal part of the Estonia project, a colleague, a historian by profession, joined me to visit the site of one of our projects: an Estonian psychologist colleague who has, since the completion of our project, become a psychoanalyst noticed that I had, in the six years he had come to know me, visited mass grave sites from Lithuania through Latvia to St. Petersburg, whenever I had some down time from the main project. Accordingly, he was intrigued. He added one more site for me to visit. This time the mass grave site was only a few miles away. The three of us spent one afternoon at this grave site that is the home of some 2000 Jewish souls. My historian colleague, who was Jewish, was quiet throughout the two-hour visit. However, after dinner, he unleashed his rage upon me as follows: "What have we done all these years in Estonia. Nothing!" He was palpably hurting. The visit to the mass grave site had caused him to have a delayed reaction. I could see it. I could hear his agony. I was quiet. I sat with him for some 40 minutes after our late dinner as he tried to diminish all that we had accomplished in Estonia. He had to destroy all our efforts. His tirade was so dissonant with his own previous assessment of our work, and my own, that I had to *be there* for him as he regressed. I watched him work his way out of his regression. He was fine the next morning. Death and our ancestors constantly leave their traces, and we have to come to grips with the remainder of their suffering, private and public.

I began this short chapter with my favorite Deleuze quote on the fold between inside and outside fields of reference. I wanted to demonstrate the interplay between the fire outside and the quietly generative psychoanalytic work inside. In the first narrative, I could be rebuffed by the resistance of a course director who asked for help with one hand but pushed me away with the other, and I was still there to deliver the fund of knowledge her students needed to build up their skills and competencies as psychoanalytically informed psychologists. In the second narrative, Indigenous Estonian and Estonian Russian kindergarten teachers could repress the embryonic creation for a framework of one collaborative project after another, and I was still there to find a kinder, gentler means of taking them back to a prior developmental place where we were all children, once upon a time, and work our way back up. In the third narrative, the pain of visiting a Jewish mass grave site was too much for my college of Jewish origin. There, too, I had to stay alive for him to recover from his temporary regression so that we could continue with the work of evaluating the outcome of our conflict-resolution project.

Now, I will end with my favorite Freud quote from *The Future of an Illusion* (1927): "The voice of the intellect is a soft one, but it does not rest until it has gained a hearing. Ultimately, after endless *rebuffs*, it succeeds. This is one of the few points which one may be optimistic about the future of mankind" (p. 53; emphasis added).

In short, the *discipline* of presiding over analytic work, inside or outside the consulting room, with the multiplicity of attitudinal, conceptual, and application tools that are available to us, can carry over into the design and implementation of group projects. We can succeed if we could see the anxiety behind the defensive rejection and the secondary interference of defense used to ward off the anxiety about change. For example, if the kindergarten teachers changed their view of the other as a historical enemy, they may have to give up long-held views of themselves and of the other.

Change is hard work. Here, meaningful change would require Indigenous Estonians to modify hatred towards their enemies who had repressed them for decades. As practitioners, we also have to come to grips with the psychic pain and associative links, ancestral or otherwise, that are activated in us while we endeavor to do our best work.

Reference

Deleuze, G. (1988). *Foucault*. London & New York: Continuum Press (Orig. 1986).

Freud, S. (1927). The future of an illusion. In *Standard Edition*, Volume 21, pp. 3–56. London: Hogarth Press, 1961.

Mearshimer, J. J. (2001). *The Tragedy of Great Power Politics*. Chicago: University of Chicago Press.

Chapter 13

Emancipation From Institutionalization

A Case Study on Transgenerational Hauntings. Edward T. Novak

Transgenerational Hauntings

The recent resurgence in attention to transgenerational trauma theories has influenced my clinical use of transactional analysis relative to the transmission of transgenerational traumas. Transgenerational trauma, or, as Apprey (2014) has suggested, transgenerational hauntings, has become a focus of concentration within the transactional analysis community (Noriega, 2004; Hargaden, 2016; Novak, 2014), including a transgenerational trauma theme issue of the *Transactional Analysis Journal* (2019).

Berne (1972) also addressed transgenerational phenomena, referring to "Ancestral Influences" (page 66), and detailed how the ancestors of a child, especially grandparents, influence the ways a child views him- or herself and how this contributes to script development. Berne added, "The most intricate part of script analysis in clinical practice is tracing back the influences of the grandparents" (p. 288).

This chapter details the history and working through of one man's transgenerational hauntings from birth to middle age. The case makes use of historical reports, clinical observations, and transgenerational and transactional analysis theories in order to provide a more complete view of the client's treatment. The case is presented in the hopes of adding to our clinical perspectives around the ways to look for and work with transgenerational hauntings within the therapeutic encounter.

In the case, I refer to the client using three names: the Boy, the Man, and the Client. These terms are used to provide the reader with a sense of where specific thoughts, feelings, or behaviors may have originated or where they seem held within this individual's psyche or body.

DOI: 10.4324/9781003389026-14

Institutional Refuge

I characterize this Client's work and journey as a saga, as it is indeed a long story, a heroic journey that begins in the Client's childhood. This saga has all the ingredients of a theoretical-based transgenerational haunting with the messenger Boy being asked to accept and run an errand (Apprey, 2014) for his family, primarily both his mother and her mother. However, I must note that the Boy's willingness to accept the errand was more out of desperation rather than heroism.

The Boy's and, later in life, the Man's entire existence was a race against two rather different but inevitable outcomes in the form of institutionalization. One ending would be a mental institution, the other prison. Neither of these institutions were exactly the ending one might want to fantasize for their life script (Berne, 1972). Yet this Client spent all of his childhood and most of his adulthood trapped between these two inevitable outcomes of a tragic script.

The Client's tragic script became even more tragic with the addition of a third possible ending: suicide. The Client's obsession with suicide seemed a natural and necessary option given his impossible circumstance. His suicide escape hatch seemed to help him deal with the madness of waiting for a possible imprisonment for a crime he was charged with but never committed. The crime was the sexual assault of his mother when he was between the ages or four and six. How a boy could be accused of such an impossible crime will be revealed as we listen to the Client's history.

This Boy's saga began way before his accused crime of sexual assault and even prior to his birth. The setting was a small town near Pittsburgh, Pennsylvania, in 1937. A mother gave birth to a beautiful daughter, the third of her children. Within the daughter's first year of life, the mother contracted tuberculosis (TB) and was whisked away to a sanitarium, an institution. Both the mother's TB and her institutionalization were to be kept secret, as the fears of tuberculosis would have created social rejection for her children.

Almost every detail the Boy learned about his mother's childhood was acquired through listening to stories she would tell both him and his sister over the course of their childhoods. Their mother spoke of her childhood pain over the unbearable loss of her mother, who "Was taken to a place where all the crazy people were put." Although sanitariums treat chronic disease, they were often confused for insane asylums. Apparently, this confusion was also embedded into the family biography. Despite the sanitarium being defined as a place that had "A bunch of crazy people walking around," the hospital was also said to have been a rather lovely place with landscaped grounds to walk about and loving doctors and nurses to take care of the patients.

The Boy and his sister also learned that their mother's only contact with her institutionalized mother between the ages 12 months and 13 years of age were sporadic monthly visits to the sanitarium. The visits included a strict policy of no physical contact. The three children and their mother would gaze at one another through a large glass window. Apparently, the children found these visits "confusing and scary." One can only imagine what it was like for these three children to be afraid of their own mother, a woman they hardly even knew.

Tuberculous took the mother's life when her daughter was 13 years old. Only the mother's husband attended the funeral. The family biography recorded this day as one where the father came home from his wife's funeral to the sight of his three children playing the radio and dancing, oblivious to the gravity of what had happened. In deeper reflection, perhaps this was the defense of three teenagers faced with the physical death of a mother who was in many ways already a ghost to them.

In her telling and retelling of the early separation and loss of her own mother, the Boy's mother was looking toward both him and his sister for witnessing they could not provide. The mother was also hoping they could provide relief from the abandonment and pain she carried, but they failed in this implicit request as well.

As therapists, we can bear witness to this woman's pain. This woman's mother essentially became a living ghost when the woman was an infant. We can imagine many clinical ways of thinking of her childhood from attachment issues to trauma. We can image what an absence of physical contact with a mother would have done to this woman. We can imagine her touching the glass that both separated and protected her from mother. We can even envision her mother looking out the second-story window and waving goodbye to her and her brothers, the children she could not mother.

But for the Boy, these narratives often proved more confusing to his developing mind than heartbreaking. Perhaps even in those early years the Boy's psyche was defending against this family's unspeakable losses.

Unconsciously, these narratives were being ingested into his own psyche and script formation, and two transgenerational themes became embedded in his family protocol. One was that family members were in danger of living in mental institutions. The second was that such matters needed to be kept secret.

The Daughter Becomes a Mother, More Secrets

Returning to the family history. In 1962 the motherless daughter has grown up, moved away, marries, and has her first child, a daughter. Ten months later she becomes pregnant with her second child, the Boy. The Boy's pregnancy was unplanned and unwanted. The story of the Boy's conception was narrated as thus, "When I found out I was pregnant with you, I was so mad at your father I could have killed him."

If the Boy's conception was untimely and infuriating, the mother's nine months of carrying him did nothing but add to her hatred and her misery over his existence. While pregnant with the Boy, her issues with chronic back pain degenerated even further, creating a herniated disk. This type of pain while pregnant would have been challenging for a well-grounded parent, let alone a mother barely hanging onto her own sanity during an unwanted pregnancy. In addition, having moved three hours away from her hometown, any limited support network of family or friends she had back home was now unavailable to her.

The Boy's birth story followed a narrative similar to his unplanned and unwanted creation story. Within his birth story, one can hear the hauntings of his mother's infancy and her relationship with her own mother. "When you were born, the nurse held you in front of me and cheerfully, said, 'Would you like to hold your baby boy?' I told her, 'No, I'm too tired, just put him in the nursery and I'll hold him tomorrow'."

At this point, the family narrative includes yet another form of institutionalization, with the child being placed into a nursery rather than loving parental arms.

Following the Boy's birth, the mother continued to experience unbearable pain and was almost certainly suffering from postpartum depression, if not psychosis. Her ability to take care of both a young daughter, now one and a half years old, along with this new infant would have been severely limited and almost impossible.

For the first nine months of the Boy's life, his mother was often taken to the same hospital as his birth for disk treatments. These were overnight stays where she would be placed in traction, a procedure where pulleys and weights were used in attempts to place tension on the lower vertebrae in hopes of stabilizing the region. These procedures proved ineffective, and the mother eventually opted to undergo the painful and invasive disk procedure of that time.

In the family biography the Boy's pregnancy is listed as the *cause* of the mother's back issues and surgery. Berne (1972) wrote of what he termed "The Torn Mother Script" (p. 77). He defined the foundation of this script as the mother telling the child that she has been sickly ever since he was born or, in a more vicious form, that she was so badly torn by his birth that she has never been the same. His reaction, and his script, is based on his own observations in the matter (p. 77).

This Boy would spend the rest of his life observing a mother who appeared destroyed by his birth.

At the time of this surgery, the Boy and his sister were taken to their paternal grandparents' home three hours away, where they spent approximately five months. The family biography includes a phrase that, "the Boy left home crawling and he came back walking."

Beyond keeping the two children alive, the grandparents' involvement with the children was limited. These were not loving grandparents, nor had they been loving parents. The family history includes a "humorous" fact that the back heads of all four sons were flat due to extensive crib time and not being held often as infants.

The Boy was 13 months old when he and his sister returned home. The repeated narrative from his mother that seemed to echo back to her own history, which was always told without feeling, was that not only did the Boy not recognize her but, "He ran away from her, frightened, and hid behind the couch."

The following year and a half of this Boy's life would find him placed back in the hospital of his birth seven times. These institutionalizations were not because of TB but because of another respiratory issue, asthma. This was the Boy's somatic response to his abandonment from his primary care objects.

Years later while in therapy and in search for answers around his childhood asthma, the Man was able to retrieve his hospital records on microfilm. His childhood records were secured for him by his wife. The Boy grew up and married a doctor who just so happened to work in the hospital of both his birth and his infant admissions.

The hospital notes were enlightening and validated many of his somatic memories of his early trauma. They included one entry dated December 24, 1965, where, had it not been for the intervention of a respiratory specialist in the late hours of the night, the Boy would have died from an acute asthma attack. These notes also helped confirm that, tragically for the infant Boy, his hospitalizations may have been his first felt experience of being cared for. The mother's report that "good doctors and nice nurses took care of you" seemed eerily reminiscent of the words used to describe her own mother's stay in the sanitarium.

The institutional caretaking theme was also expressed in the mother's blunt admission that, "Your father and I couldn't bear taking care of you when you were sick." She often added, "You should have died" with a period behind the word died, rather than a comma followed by "and I'm so glad you didn't."

This portion of the family biography has three major conclusions not missed by the astute Boy that contributed to his script formation (Berne, 1972). First, a hospital institution saved his life. Second, his parents were not able to keep him alive. Third, he should have died, contributing to a "don't exist" injunction (Goulding & Goulding, 1976), which haunted the Boy well into his middle age.

We could spend pages speaking to this Client's work in therapy after he discovered the injunction "Don't exist" and his counterinjunction, "It is okay for me to exist if I don't have any needs and take care of everyone else." However, the thread we are following is institutional hauntings, and we will continue along on that thread.

Institutions of Foster Homes and Prisons

Returning to the mother's childhood history: the unimaginable loss of her mother in infancy would have created lifelong issues for her even in a supportive and stable home environment. Sadly, her home environment was torturous.

She and her two brothers were raised, or perhaps we should say kept alive, by a father who worked all day and drank at bars late into the evening. The children were generally home alone and left to essentially take care of themselves.

When she spoke privately to her son, the Boy heard hints that she was sexually abused by her father. This abuse had been kept secret with the threat that if anyone found out, she would be taken away and placed in a foster home where she would never see her father, brothers, or mother ever again. One can only imagine the terror and despair this young girl carried within her traumas and the secrets.

Her father's threats were convincing, and she never told anyone about his molestation of her. In this way, her abuse history became a mystified secret (Apprey, 2019) within the family. Apprey notes how the mystification of secrets is accomplished through. "the lies families tell to conceal a secret for a defensive purpose in order to mitigate anxiety" (p. 340).

Apprey (2019) then notes how Abraham (1975/1994) believes the mystification of secrets subsequently feeds pathological formations (p. 340). In this case the pathological formation included a reverence of the father that continued into future generations. The family folklore became the grandfather was a noble gentleman who raised three children on his own. The pathological narrative omitted both his alcoholism and sexual abuse of his daughter.

Transgenerational trauma theory, including transactional analysis ideas of the hot potato (English, 1969), would predict the mystified family secrets would need to be passed on to someone who could decode and translate these experiences into a revised family biography. Almost predictably, the responsibility for revising this family's biography would fall on the first-born son to this woman., the Boy.

Apprey (2014) describes the process as "infusion" (p. 16) or "injection" (p. 24). In this case, the mother's trauma was injected into her son. The Boy was ages four to six when he was told in great detail by his mother of her sexual abuse. However, there would be a 40-year delay, or Apprey's (2019) term, "deferral" (p. 340), in his ability to decode and translate this information as his mother communicated her sexual abuse through body and touch, not words.

This abuse was a replication of the abuse the mother had endured from her own father. The mother would choreograph the Boy as to how he should engage with her body that imitated ways her father had abused her.

For the Boy, given the absence of loving physical connections with his mother, these physical moments were sanctified experiences, filled with a sense of meeting and knowing his mother for the first time. He was unaware that loving and intimate touch toward his mother could be anything but blissful. However, his full immersion into an "harmonious interpenetrating mix-up" (Balint, 1979, p. 66) was abruptly destroyed as his mother shifted from pleasure to outrage. She told him what he did to her was wrong and that she had not wanted him to touch her in those ways.

In what had to have been an almost direct replay of her interactions with her own father, the Boy was threated that if anyone found out what he had done to her, the police would take him away to a foster home, or jail, where he would never see any of his family again.

The Boy unconsciously dealt with this abuse and his confusion of touch through the use of dissociation. The experiences of sexual molestation from his mother became buried deep within the Boy's psyche, only to make an overwhelming return in his 40s.

What did remain was a belief that one day he was going to be unwillingly institutionalized. Now, there could be one of three possible institutional outcomes: a hospital, a foster home, or prison. When he turned 18, foster homes were no longer an option, and he was left the options of hospital or prison.

Fate would decide which one of these would be his tragic script ending. Would he go crazy and end up in a mental institution? A place with clean white sheets, smiling nurses, three meals a day, and beautiful grounds to walk around. This reflected his fantasy for a good mother in the form of a mental hospital. Would he be arrested and placed in a prison for crimes he was found guilty of but did not commit? Prison became an institution of punishment not only for his sexual crimes but also for his birth that crippled his mother. He was in fact a "Villain" (Berne, 1972, p. 77).

Living with this inevitable fate created unbearable anxiety for the Boy, and later Man. Because this part of his history had been dissociated, his thoughts and fears of forced placement into an institution felt psychotic. The belief in an institutional script ending became an organizing principle in his psyche.

Suicidal fantasies also became a part of his daily thoughts. The escape hatch of suicide allowed for a way to rid himself of the unbearable anticipatory panic around an interminable life of unjust incarceration if that was his fate. However, this was certainly not the hoped-for option, and as the Boy became a Man, he looked for ways to alter his fate.

Turning Fate Into a Destiny

The Man was resilient and worked unconsciously to find an alternative institution to those which fate had in store for him. At age 17 he was in the throes of his first of many non-psychotic breakdowns (Bollas, 2013) that went unrecognized by those around him. However, he sensed he was in big trouble and at risk of leading a tragic adult life, if he didn't kill himself first.

In what turned out to be a life-changing, and saving, decision, the young Man decided to metaphorically pink slip himself into not one but two of the finest institutions his Catholic upbringing could imagine. This moment also marked a shift from fate to destiny (Bollas, 1989). The young Man institutionalized himself into a religious order, the Brothers of Holy Cross, and their institutional home base, the University of Notre Dame.

Notre Dame was a different experience for this young Man than most college students. His college life was not experienced in a dormitory but within the type of institutional living religious life provides. The young Man was educated and nurtured by remarkable men of faith. The Holy Cross Brothers became the second experience of being cared for within an institutional family. This institution appeared to be a true oasis and rescue from his haunted fate.

However, despite a strong desire and commitment to remain a part of the religious order, spiritual calling was neither fate nor destiny for this young Man, and he would have to move on beyond the security these men had provided. Their love and knowledge he would, however, take with him.

When this case was consulted with Maurice Apprey (Personal communication, May 31, 2019), Apprey referred to the young Man's decision to join the Holy Cross Brothers at Notre Dame as an important "false start" in working through his errand and reclaiming his life. The saga of an errand is not a linear journey. False starts and wrong turns are inevitable. However, each false start and wrong turn creates more insights and understanding of both family and self if self-analyzed. Eventually, these non-linear experiences create a scatterplot that points the person in the necessary direction, where hauntings are revealed and life scripts changed.

Despite this and other false starts, the young Man was able to achieve a great deal, including a loving long-term marriage and raising a wonderful son. Internally, however, he remained haunted. This was the type of haunting Berne (1972) described of individuals who do not reside within their own secret garden. Rather, perhaps like ghost themselves, they wander, "wistfully outside their own walls" (p. 130).

A Life Haunted by Institutions

In his late 20s, the Man entered into his first therapy based in transactional analysis theory. Over a decade of work in that treatment found him exploring his life script, injunctions such as "don't exist," counterinjunctions such as "it's okay if I'm alive as long as I help people," and his suicide escape hatch.

The Man also entered intensive body work and body psychotherapy to reclaim his stolen body and a new belief that touching another human being would not have him falsely accused of sexual abuse and imprisoned. These issues required decades of body therapy and proved to be some of his most difficult work, given so much of his embodied traumas occurred in early childhood.

What made this Client's case difficult to understand was despite all the work he achieved, he continued to report,

> I don't feel the way someone should feel after all this good work. I should feel better inside, less hateful of myself and fearful of going crazy and into a mental hospital. I know I won't end up in prison anymore, but I can't get rid of the belief I'm going to go crazy and end up in a mental hospital.

The problem, and transformation, would soon be revealed to him within a transgenerational haunting. It was a seminar on September 7, 2019, where an angelic ghost, became transformed into a family ancestor.

The Boy Meets His Grandma for the First Time

I was attending a much-anticipated seminar on transgenerational trauma conducted by Maurice Apprey and Adrienne Harris when Dr. Harris presented a case illustration on a three-generational haunting. She and Dr. Apprey had been emphasizing that in working with transgenerational trauma, it is not enough to go back two generations in treatment, those being client and parents. Rather, she and Apprey were advocating that therapists try to have clients take them back to at least a third generation, grandparents.

This was in line with Berne's (1972) belief that a script is passed from grandparent to parent to child. He called this process "The Family Parade" (p. 283). Later, James (1984) wrote an article addressing this issue titled "Grandparents and the Family Script Parade" (p. 18).

I began to apply a three-generational model and Dr. Harris's case to my clinical work. I thought of my work with a female client I had been seeing for a number of years. On a clean sheet of paper, I attempted to detail and diagram her hauntings using Dr. Apprey's model. However, I found Dr. Apprey's intricate model of analyzing transgenerational material more complicated than I could duplicate. Nonetheless, what I could make use of in his model certainly affirmed the path the client and I were on in her treatment. I was trying to fit the case into theory rather than theory into the case. This is an example of where a theory-driven process may overshadow clinical observations.

I shifted my thoughts to another case, the Boy. I also suspended my attempts to replicate Dr. Apprey's use of his theory. I opted for a more generalized approach, blending his theoretical model with transactional analysis constructs and an informal diagram of ego states. From within Apprey's model, I reflected on the institutionalized woman in the Boy's history. She was a ghost who had taken on a more ethereal identity in the family biography. The Boy had grown up with a vision of her as an angelic figure. He had often fantasized of her standing in a clean white hospital gown, with beautiful long black hair, and sadly but regally waving to her three children from a second-story sanitarium window. The family biography had always described her as a beautiful woman. There has never been a reason to believe this was untrue.

I took these reflections and worked with them in a more transactional analytic frame. As I thought of this Boy and his work as an Adult Client, I wrote on my note page, "grandma–mother–boy." I now had a transgenerational model of P-A-C. I began to explore possible similarities between the three of them to see if I could identify any ghosts or hauntings I may have missed or not fully developed about the Boy and his transgenerational history.

At that moment in the seminar, two thoughts began to formulate in my mind that forever changed the trajectory of my life. I sat there not as the Boy, not as the Man, and not even as the Client I had been in therapy for over 30 years but as a therapist. At that moment I was in a therapeutic self-analytic space not inhabited by ghosts.

From this observing ego, I was recognizing my own omission of not going back three generations in my own maternal history. I became more curious about the P on the diagram, my mother's mother. In that moment I discovered two distinct aspects of my transgenerational history. First, I realized that I knew almost nothing about my maternal grandmother, other than that she was confined to a sanitarium for 12 years with TB.

As I reflected on this woman's life with newfound curiosity and empathy, a second insight became available to me. I sat there silently repeating one word I had written in my notes, "Grandma." I was 56 years old, and until that specific moment I had never seen or addressed this beautiful and tragic figure as "my Grandma."

I was finally understanding my intense fears of going crazy and being placed in a mental institution were not merely my psychotic creations. Rather they were part of an unconscious family edict that one day Grandma-mother-and I would all be reunited in a sanatorium. I was also now able to discriminate between the beliefs held by the "there and then Boy," and the "here and now Man."

My mother had received, in transactional analysis terms, an institutional script, in Apprey's terms, a haunting. This script and haunting had been transmitted to her by each parent through different behaviors and messages. My mother then continued "the family parade of scripts" (James, 1984, p. 19) passing on the institutional script to me.

As stated earlier, Berne (1972) had noted the importance of grandparents relative to script and script analysis. James (1984) wrote of how even "a grandparent 'in absentia' may feel like a ghost, exerting either a positive or negative influence on the grandchildren through the parents" (p. 21). For years my error had been to overlook her influence, assuming that because my maternal grandmother was deceased, her impact on my psyche and script had been minimal.

With an awareness of my maternal grandmother's influence, I could now bring in another portion of Apprey's model. After years of trying to fully grasp his theories around a pluperfect errand, they were now not only making sense; they were unfolding right in front of me. I could now link his theory to both my family biography and transactional analysis script theory.

Apprey's (2014) quote, "What happens now shall have already happened" (p. 16) came to mind. Although my grandmother was dead, in the world of the psyche, past, present, and future can all be one. Until this seminar, I had viewed the origins of my script exclusively within a haunted past. I never had considered my grandmother could be part of my haunted present.

This meant that in my psyche, there was a world where my grandmother was still locked away in a sanatorium. My mother had longed for reunion with her mother, and I was unconsciously including myself in that reunion. Given my grandmother's illness, this reunion could only take place in mental hospital. I assume my sister was also a part of this reunion, but for the purpose of this chapter, I won't move into that thread of processing.

This unconscious transmission of this reunion had created the following internal conflict. For years, one part of my internal self, the Adult, was convinced I would never end up in a sanatorium. At the same time, another part of my self, the Boy, was convinced that such an outcome was both necessary and inevitable. Worse, if he didn't go crazy and end up in a mental hospital, prison would be his fate. It is no wonder a suicide escape hatch seemed a necessary option.

As past, present, and future could now be seen separately, I could live within a conscious realization that my grandmother and my mother were both dead and therefore I could not possibly reunite with them in a sanatorium or mental hospital. I was now free to begin to explore a life not haunted by a fear of institutionalization.

Way Stations and the Expansive Reach of Hauntings

The transformations that followed my emancipation occurred at speeds that are generally not possible in mental health treatment. However, I have also witnessed these remarkable shifts in clients after they emancipate from transgenerational hauntings and scripts. Following emancipation, the client's script is no longer a mandate. This allows for psychic reconfiguration and transformation that naturally leads then to external changes in the client's relationships and lived experience.

For me, I had achieved an emancipation I was unaware I had ever needed. I was now living without an internal fear of going crazy and being placed in an institution or in prison for a sexual crime I was falsely accused of committing.

I had also liberated my grandmother from the sanitarium she was still locked-up in within my family's and my psyche. She was now an ancestor rather than an angelic figure.

I also was able to revisit my own mother's unconscious lifelong search for reunion with her institutionalized mother. Hospitals and doctors were an integral part my childhood. For my mother, they were a symbolic substitute for her own mother.

My mother would often schedule doctor visits for minor, if not nonexistent, issues. This intensified in her later years as her health began to decline and she received many precautionary hospital admissions. These admissions generally resulted in a clean bill of health for a woman her age. I had always remarked that my mother would have lived in a hospital if she could. That comment was now actually making sense.

I could also understand why I too had unconsciously used mental institutions as an organizing principle in my psyche. However, unlike my mother, I was trying to replace my inevitable fate of a mandated institutionalization with a more destiny-filled choice. This included my early adult decision to enter the religious life.

Prior to the seminar with Dr. Apprey and Dr. Harris, I had scheduled a trip to Notre Dame for the following weekend. My wife and I were to spend the weekend with my Holy Cross family. Late into our first evening, I decided to take a solitary walk around the campus for some reflective alone time.

The walk was enlightening, as I could sense that Notre Dame no longer needed to be a waystation, a place that provided me safe harbor until I ultimately was admitted to a sanitarium. For the first time in over 30 years, I was able to walk the hallowed grounds of the university without needing to feel the university as a symbolic mother and waystation for a journey towards a sanitarium.

This recognition and transformation opened up my ability to see other places that I had unconsciously converted into psychic waystations. Many of these places will remain important aspects of my life, but they are no longer waystations on a journey toward a tragic script end within an institutionalization. As my fears of mental hospitals and prisons evaporated, so did the need for a suicide escape hatch.

Shooting the Messenger—From Emancipation to Excommunication

In my work with clients, I have found that many errands end not only with emancipation but excommunication from the family. This should not be that surprising when we understand many family systems are strongly invested in maintaining a happier but often fictional family biography that necessitates the concealment of family secrets through their mystification.

A family member who retrieves secrets from within the sedimentations of family history (Apprey, 2019) and becomes an intermediator between the family biography and their revised autobiography is often not received with a hero's or heroine's welcome. Rather, there can be aggressive attempts to coerce them into silence around their discoveries. Many times, there is retribution for uncovering and revealing family secrets. The retribution can include attacks on the messenger's credibility or sanity, or even excommunication.

Often a family's level of acceptance of biographical revisions depends upon whether the trauma and secret originated within the family or if they were external to the family system. Traumas created outside the family system, such as wars and natural disasters, may evoke less family resistance to examining recovered transgenerational traumas than trauma that originates in the form of abuse within the family.

Part of the work in therapy is processing with the client their thoughts on how to proceed in the light of this new information. Exploring the possible family responses to the client must be factored into the therapy as part of the working through of the transgenerational hauntings. More important than the family's response to revelations discovered within the completed errand will be the way the client can make peace and use of his or her discoveries.

Epilogue—Making Peace With Ghosts

In this chapter, I have attempted to cover over 80 years of family history and ghosts that had haunted me at both psychic and embodied levels. In presenting my personal history as a clinical case, I have attempted to provide the reader with the type of psychic space that is generally available when reflecting on a clinical case. Through the concealment of my identity in the case, it was my hope the reader could immerse him- or herself into the case material in a more unbiased fashion.

My 30-year saga with four different therapists, countless massage therapists, and body workers helped me to eventually emancipate from my ancestral hauntings and also reclaim my stolen body.

In understanding my own family constellation and entanglements (Welford, 2019) and then making peace with my transgenerational hauntings, I have be able to both transform and reconfigure my relationship with my mother within various ego and self-states. Rather than a more integrated transformation, each state seems to have been reconfigured in ways that correspond to that specific part of my life experience. This is because I have had multiple and different relational experiences with my mother, dependent in part on her own moods, ego states, and mental health.

The following is my brief attempt at detailing how I experience and relate to my mother from within my own various ego and self-states, in hopes that clients and therapist can use my experience as both example and reference.

Within my experience as the Boy, or Child, ego, I have always related to my mother with love, longing, and fear. This is generally the relational experience of a child with a disorganized parental attachment (Hesse & Main, 1999). The ability to split off the good from the bad and then blame myself for the bad served me well in order to retain a necessary attachment to her. But I paid a high price for this attachment.

Within this Child ego, I have never fully understood how the charges of sexual assault were dropped and forgotten. This is evidenced by my occasional regression back into fear and distrust of touch. However, within an Adult perspective of my history, these instances have become acute moments rather than a continued lifelong pattern. And if my mother were alive today, this Child part of my self would still love her deeply and be deeply terrified of her as well.

From my Adult ego state, I viewed my mother as a perpetrator of crimes on a young boy that merited imprisonment. While I now can experience moments of empathy for her own tragic life and childhood, her abuse and hatred of me make a more sustained empathic position difficult. To be the victimized, empathizer, and forgiver is a task too heavy for this specific part of myself to execute. In addition, a more objective position in my Adult psyche is necessary for when my Child ego is creating connections with Mom. This Adult part of my self provides a form of *psychic supervised visitation* that ensures protection from the trauma memories of the past.

From my perspective as therapist, my mother was not a perpetrator of crimes on a young boy that merited imprisonment. My mother was both victim and perpetrator, or more accurately, both abused girl and psychotic mother. I have little doubt my mother's early history was horrific and unbearable and that she was never able to recovery from such an impossible beginning of life. Knowing the characteristics of trauma and dissociation, I am certain my mother led a haunted existence.

The absence of loving physical contact from my mother certainly can be traced back to her own relationship with a mother whose physical proximity to her could have been deadly. The sexual abuse from her father would have added multiple layers to her anxieties and confusions of touch that were then enacted and transmitted into me. From my therapeutic perspective, I have empathy for many people, my grandmother, my sister, myself, and my mother, especially for her childhood.

In working with transgenerational hauntings, each therapist will make the use of theory in their clinical work with clients differently, based upon the needs of each specific client. Making use of transgenerational theories, being curious about the client's family hauntings, and providing safe space for deeper exploration of them can lead to unimagined psychic transformations for the client.

References

Abraham, N. (1994). Notes on the phantom: A complement to Freud's metapsychology. In *The Shell and the Kernel: Renewals of Psychoanalysis*, eds. N. Abraham & M. Torok, Volume 1, pp. 171–176. Chicago & London: The University of Chicago Press (Orig. 1975).

Apprey, M. (2014). A pluperfect errand: A turbulent return to beginnings in the transgenerational transmission of destructive aggression. *Free Associations*, 15(2): 16–29.

Apprey, M., interviewed by Cornell, W. F. (2019). Scripting inhabitations of unwelcome guests, hosts, and ghosts: Unpacking elements that constitute transgenerational haunting. *Transactional Analysis Journal*: 339–351. https://doi.org/10.1080/03621537.2019.1650234

Balint, M. (1979). *The Basic Fault: Therapeutic Aspects of Regression*. London & New York: Tavistock Publications.

Berne, E. (1972). *What Do You Say after You Say Hello? The Psychology of Human Destiny*. New York, NY: Grove Press.

Bollas, C. (1989). *Forces of Destiny: Psychoanalysis and Human Idiom*. Northvale, NJ: Jason Aronson.

Bollas, C. (2013). *Catch them before They Fall: The Psychoanalysis of Breakdown*. London: Routledge.

English, F. (1969). Episcript and the "hot potato" game. *Transactional Analysis Bulletin*, 8(32): 77–82.

Goulding, M. & Goulding, R. (1976). Injunctions, decisions, and redecisions. *Transactional Analysis Journal*, 6(1): 41–48. http://doi.org/10.1177/036215377600 600110

Hargaden, H. (2016). The role of the imagination in an analysis of unconscious relatedness. *Transactional Analysis Journal*, 46(4): 311–321.

Hesse, E. & Main, M. (1999). Second-generation effects of unresolved trauma in nonmaltreating parents: Dissociated, frightened, and threatening parental behavior. *Psychoanalytic Inquiry*, 19(4): 481–540.

James, J. (1984). Grandparents and the family script parade. *Transactional Analysis Journal*, 14(1): 18–28. http://doi.org/10.1177/036215378401400104

Noriega, G. (2004). Codependence: A transgenerational script. *Transactional Analysis Journal*, 34: 312–322.

Novak, E. (2014). When relief replaces loss: Parental hatred that forecloses loving attachment. *Transactional Analysis Journal*, 44(4): 255–267.

Welford, E. (2019). Healing the fallout from transgenerational trauma: Supporting clients in making peace with their history. *Transactional Analysis Journal*, 49(4): 324–338.

Chapter 14

Thrown

A Personal Narrative of Psychoanalysis and Toxic Errands.
William F. Cornell

For more than a decade, Maurice Apprey has been a psychoanalytic mentor in my professional development. What was quite unexpected, however, were the ways in which his writing and knowing him have affected my personal life. The chapters that fill this book bring to life the complex and often troubling terrain of the unconscious embeddedness of the tragedies and secrets of generations past on those living in the present.

In addition to my two psychoanalyses over the course of 25 years—each of which significantly fostered a psychic and interpersonal freedom in my later years—it has been through my readings of and study with Maurice Apprey regarding transgenerational haunting that I could more fully understand the infusion and impact of death and despair within the earlier generations on my own psyche, creating—perhaps even before my birth—the urgency and psychic demand that Apprey frames as transgenerational haunting:

> In transgenerational haunting, then, a contemporary generation is unwittingly possessed by an earlier generation. The possession preserves history, but in a poisonous, unmetabolized version.
>
> (2003, p. 12)

This chapter is an effort to present my own psychoanalyses as a case study presented and then re-examined and deepened through the lens of transgenerational haunting.

On Being *"Thrown"*

Apprey, through his unique interweaving of psychoanalysis and phenomenology, speaks of how the infant, often even before birth, is *thrown* into

DOI: 10.4324/9781003389026-15

roles and functions to fulfill the unconscious needs and fantasies of the prior generations. We are each at birth "thrown" into a particular body and psyche, during a very particular place in time in history and culture within particular family circumstances, that lay the foundation of our unconscious experience and organization. So, from the very start, one may have no choice and little awareness of this underlying operational system.

In Apprey's conception, a transgenerational "errand" is sent from a dead generation into the psyche of a living generation, such that someone else's intentionality will or has come to be made one's own:

> At the outset something is *injected* from an anterior source; that something is *housed* in a hospitable place for storage for an indeterminate time; that same something is *suspended*; that something that is stored in this time warp carries *a mandate for an errand* to be carried out. Upon the mandate's urgent/voluntary reception, the subject awaits a suitable new object to reawaken the project so that that pro-ject *can return to a public space away from a haunt,* as it were. By this time the subject shall have lost sight of who sent whom. *Active and passive have by now become interchangeable.*
>
> (p. 76, this volume)

Apprey (2003) elaborates on the nature of these qualities of injection and mandate by drawing upon Laplanche's differentiation of implantation and intromission and in so doing seeks to capture the difference between the subjective experience of more neurotic defenses and those which are the product of transgenerational *haunting*:

> According to Laplanche, then, implantation allows the injured party to actively take things up as well as translate or repress the injury. Intromission, however, forecloses translation or transformation. Intromission renders the injury resistant to change. His words are worth echoing again and again: *intromission short-circuits differentiation and "puts into the interior an element resistant to all metabolization."*
>
> (p. 10, emphasis in the original)

Herein, I think, lies the quality of being possessed that is so central to Apprey's articulation of transgenerational *haunting*, a realm inhabited by the tattered ghosts and phantoms of times and loved ones long past.

Transgenerational Haunting

In his articulation of *haunting*, Apprey brings a unique and important voice to the psychoanalysis of unconscious, intergenerational communications. These traumatized, transgenerational personages may be full of violence, despair, and hopelessness, but they may also be messengers, carriers, of insistent, urgent hopes and demands. Such relentless, unconsciously driven pressures are what Apprey names unconscious "errands":

> To be precise, sometimes when we think we have an active project, we have actually been sent on *an errand.* Here, an ancestral project, founded, and foundered, placed and misplaced, long ago, still lingers but in the hands of a new a suitable carrier. Past and present change places; subject and object change places . . . sometimes, *the moment I am named I have been sent off packing on a journey, on an errand and at a parent's or grandparent's bidding.* Whose errand is it? Whose bidding is it? Whose journey is it? *Who is held hostage on the errand? Who is mis-taken?*
>
> (2019, p. 349, emphasis in the original)

These are the ghosts who carry the knowing of unbearable tragedies, just as they are spirits of hope for the future, *unconscious demands* upon subsequent generations who have a chance at better lives. Apprey (1999) argues, "I want to suggest that the fact of history has an *urgency*; it cries out for recognition and meaning" (p. 135). The urgency of the unconscious, received injuries and "errands" (p. 136) are conveyed from one generation to the next, awaiting detoxification so as to return freedom to those who have been inhabited by the errand.

Through his work with transgenerational haunting Apprey (2003, 2006) has developed a model that facilitates the analysis of the roots, the force, and the meaning of these errands. An essential part of the analytic work is then to differentiate the future incorporated as *errand* built upon generational debris from the desires and possibilities of the emerging psyche of a growing child (or struggling patient) with an intentionality of their own. In my reading and experience of Apprey's analytic sensibility is a profound respect for the richness and meanings of the unlived "futures" that enliven the transgenerational errands while creating—instilling—the psychic space for individuation and differentiation.

Shadows and Chasms in My Family's History

I had the good fortune to know the care of my maternal grandparents. My parents were introduced immediately after the war and soon married. Born in 1947, I was brought into the world with all the expectations of a first-born son and ushered into the manic, victorious climate of post-war America. It was then sometime after my birth that my father suffered a breakdown, a well-kept family secret, a product of my father's suffering after his return from the war. We moved into the home of my maternal grandparents. They became my primary caretakers, and it was in their arms that I knew comfort and pleasure in the earliest years of my life. But my mother then suffered two miscarriages before being able to give birth to another son and then a daughter. During that period her beloved father was fighting an intense battle against lung cancer. He lost the battle, and both my mother and grandmother collapsed into prolonged depressions. I was seven years old and still vividly recall the pall of despair that descended on the family. My father did not have the resources to help my mother (or himself) grieve.

My grandfather was a first-generation Italian immigrant, my grandmother first generation German immigrant—each the youngest of 13 children. Like immigrants of that era, while they preserved the foods and certain rituals of their places of origin, I never heard them speak their birth languages. Like so many immigrant families to America, they did not look back. What it was they were leaving, what it was they were escaping, was never discussed. They looked forward, not backward, with a determination that was both repressive and manic.

I knew my maternal grandmother's extended family very well, as most lived within a few city blocks of one another. She was a year old when her father died suddenly, leaving her mother, who spoke little English, with 13 children. Never to remarry, this young German immigrant, with the labor of the older sons and the support of the local Catholic parish, kept the family together. My grandmother volunteered all her life in that church to repay the parish for keeping her family together. But her father's sudden death marked her and the family, as did the later accidental death of a brother, a trauma that never left her. Then the death of her beloved husband before the age of 50 left her bereft. I knew my grandmother as hard-working, loyal, and depressed for most of her life, her tenderness always imbued with a loneliness.

I did not learn until many years after my grandfather's death that his was a Sicilian family brought to the United States to join a Cosa Nostra family in upstate New York. As the youngest son in the family, he opted not to join the family "business." As a result, he was cut off by the family. I had never met a member of his family until, at the age of seven, I met all these people with the same last name as my grandfather who came to his wake. He made his way in life as an uneducated, loving, devoted, and hard-working man. My maternal grandparents, father, and mother all shared hard work accompanied by silence about their internal lives.

Schwab (2010) has observed:

> People have always silenced violent histories. Some histories, collective and personal, are so violent we would not be able to live our daily lives if we did not at least temporarily silence them. . . . Too much silence, however, becomes haunting.
>
> (p. 46)

The silences that surrounded me growing up were not meant to be cruel. They were intended to be a kind of protective cushion. We learned to live in silence in the face of trouble. By the time of my own adult life, my tendency toward silence isolated me, coming to serve much more as a barrier than a cushion, often leaving me a stranger to those who cared for me.

For this chapter, I will describe three decisive moments, "scenes," from my analytic therapies which constituted major, disarming steps forward in challenging and softening my chronic characterological defenses. I will then re-examine these scenes through the lens of transgenerational haunting and the compelling, unconscious errand that had compelled me through much of my adolescence and adult life. While this errand brought me and those around me much satisfaction and accomplishment, the toxic costs on this transgenerational mission took decades to become fully known and felt.

Scene One: Parents

I had entered psychoanalysis in my early 40s struggling with a decision to leave a deeply troubled marriage while parenting three boys.

"Your entire character is founded on your determination that no one you love will ever experience loss," came the voice of my analyst from behind my head. His voice was so unusually insistent. I felt as though he were shouting in bold italics. I no longer remember clearly what it was that I'd been talking about (most likely some concern about one of my sons), but his words and tone stunned me. He went on to elaborate his unexpected pronouncement, pulling together disparate threads of past and present that I had never allowed to coalesce within my own experience so as to create meaning.

He vividly recalled the loneliness and isolation that I had endured during my mother's death at 39 while I was in college, followed by my father's death at 50 while I was struggling to craft a life as a young adult and father. His was not a cerebral interpretation but rather an emotional statement of a reality that I had fended off for more than 20 years. Yet I immediately knew the truth of his words in my bones—that I had been unconsciously determined that my sons would not have to endure loss, that somehow magically I could keep them safe. Now, my analyst declared, we could stand and face the losses of my impending divorce together. I was not alone, and my sons would not be left to fend for themselves.

My father was the third of four siblings, an older brother and sister, a younger brother. He was seven when his father died unexpectedly of a medical error. His mother quickly became more deeply involved with the man with whom she had been having an affair, leaving the bereaved kids to pretty much manage for themselves. This was not a story ever told to me by my father; his has been a bitter account of blame for their childhood poverty (although, in fact, they had been quite middle class), leaving all the ugly details out. This was the account told to me by his older sister after my father's death. Through my aunt, I learned that the family had suffered far more disturbance and rupture than my father had ever revealed. For my father and his siblings, there was never the cushion or resilience of an extended family. My father was a teenager when he fled the family in favor of World War II. The war had not been my father's only silenced trauma.

He came back a broken man from a war in which the returning soldiers were hailed as heroes. So, he endured his anguish in a silent withdrawal, doing his best to earn a living, live a decent life, and protect his children from his inner demons. Neither of my parents completed high school. My father worked in factory, did night school to gradually earn his high school diploma and ultimately some college credits, and, for extra income, repaired televisions in the basement. We rarely saw him. My mother worked at home as a seamstress and laundress. Their lives were not easy.

Encased in an anguished silence, his unspoken suffering was nevertheless passed on to his children. But the history and facts of his suffering remained unknown to them. Then a brief window into my father's anguish opened unexpectedly: I had refused induction to the draft during the Vietnam war, filing for conscientious objector status based on political rather than religious grounds. To my utter surprise, this father who rarely spoke wrote an impassioned and articulate letter to my draft board, saying that as a veteran of World War II, he could never allow a child of his to participate in any war. Yet in spite of his letter and my repeated inquiries, he refused to speak of what happened to him (or what he did) during the war, but I finally understood something about my father's suffering.

Our family, on both the maternal and paternal sides, had been scarred for generations by the sudden deaths of parents (usually the father) early in life. These families could not grieve. This is the transgenerational cauldron into which I was born and *thrown*. My mother's family tended to collapse into various forms of depressive symbioses. My father's family tended to fragment into bitter, silent isolation. Our Mom was a difficult, volatile, and quite childlike woman. Our Dad was a kind, devoted man, and all three of us siblings tended to identify with him, mirroring his patterns of silent withdrawal in the face of difficulty. As the first born and named after my father and his father, I was thrown into the errand of the manic overcoming of loss.

When my analyst made his declaration of the meaning of my character, the troubled territory of my parents' lives and my own was suddenly alive with the affect, meaning, and accompaniment, now no longer alone.

Scene Two: Siblings

At the time that I was thought my psychoanalysis was coming to a close, my analyst asked me, "Do you ever wonder how it is that while you never mention your brother or your sister, as though they have never existed, that I find them often on my mind?"

"No," was my singular reply.

"Perhaps we could wonder about it together?"

"I'm not interested. My brother and sister have never been a part of my life. Why the fuck are you bringing it up now?"

"I don't know really, it's just that I find them on my mind. And you don't seem to have them in yours. Might we wonder why my question has evoked such anger in you?"

All that I could feel was my anger in response to what I experienced as a stupid, rather ill-timed intrusion. No other answer was to come right away. I didn't even want to think about it. But now I was stuck—the life-long absence of my brother and sister in my life was now planted firmly on my mind. Gradually what I came to realize was that I had come through my analysis to a point of reaching a compassionate understanding and acceptance of my parents and their limitations. When I began to think about my brother and sister, my acceptance of my parents fell into ruins. I found myself hating my parents again, and I didn't want to do that. I had preferred to sacrifice the psychic existence of my living siblings than lose the connection I had at last forged to my deceased parents.

In keeping with my urgent errand, I was the one who—off to college—had appeared to escape the final collapse of our family. I was the one who had been able to create a good life. What little support and energy my parents had to offer, they gave to me.

Though only four years older than my brother, Gary, and six years older than my sister, Debbie, I grew up essentially as an only child. I recall having no particular interest in my siblings; I cannot recall even playing with them. Growing up in rural upstate New York, the center of my life was school, the outdoors, and my dogs. My intelligence was idealized by my teachers and parents, and I felt alive in their praise, and utterly oblivious to the "urgent errand" that I was carrying out. I lived my childhood years as though I had no siblings. I also had no close friends. All of my close relationships were with my teachers.

In my preparations for this chapter, I had hoped, wished to recall moments of intimacy with my brother and sister growing up. I could not find them. Even on the annual family trip to a camp in the Adirondack Mountains, I cannot recall actually playing with my siblings. I cannot recall taking my little brother along with me into the woods and creeks. I was never in the house any longer than I needed to be, and—rather strangely—my parents never seemed to be troubled by this. I was, perhaps, the only "trouble-free" part of their lives; I was the teacher's pet from kindergarten on and ridiculously independent from a very early age. When I was 11, we moved into a slightly larger house in town, and my father built me a bedroom in the basement with its own entrance. He told me I was old enough to come and go as I pleased. I did. There was no place for my siblings in the world of my childhood and adolescence. I never stopped moving and doing things. It appeared that I had risen above it all with stellar high school accomplishments and a full scholarship to any exceptional college.

I had been at college less than a year when the final blow to the life of my family came with my mother's diagnosis with terminal leukemia. Although I was away at college, I was deeply involved in my mother's illness through frequent letters and phone calls from my bereft parents. I knew that she would likely die. Though my brother and sister were living at home and knew that Mom was sick, my parents never told them *how* sick. Then she died suddenly as the result of a medical error. Her death was a total shock to all of us. My father collapsed in the face of it and left his younger children, then 12 and 14, to fend for themselves. I had no idea of this at the time, as no one told me. It would never have occurred to my brother or sister to call me for help or for me to call and check on them. It did not occur to me to inquire after them. I, again, escaped in a manic fleeing of the unbearable anguish on my family. I returned to college to complete my studies and prepare for graduate school. I turned to no one. I sustained myself through injecting amphetamines and heroin. This "sustenance" proved to be short lived, as I soon dropped out of college, turned to petty crimes to support myself and my habit, and ended up facing time in the Oregon penitentiary.

This time I was not left alone. My college (Reed College) learned of my plight and intervened to pay my bail, return me to school, and arrange for me to live with a passionate, left-wing family who provided a home unlike anything I had ever known. I reengaged with life and found a deep sense of belonging in this family. It is only now looking back, with Apprey's accounts of transgenerational haunting, that I can see and feel the knife edge of the toxic, urgent errand into which I had been thrown—I had, on the one hand, been invited back to my education and into a vital new family life largely as a result of my energy, intelligence, and accomplishments (which merited a second chance) while, on the other hand, I was still engaged in manic denial of the pain in my own deeply troubled self.

After college and graduate school, I started a family of my own, but I gave my brother and sister nothing of my life. I left them in the dirt.

Our father had been only 40 when he lost his beloved wife, who was then 39 and who, like his own father, died suddenly as a result of a medical error. After our mother's death, Dad's life became increasingly unbearable. I twice talked him out of shooting himself. Eight years after the death of our mother, he told me that had esophageal cancer, and he had decided to leave it untreated. He was done. Significantly, to speak to the utter depth of destructive, toxic errands, my father was then living next door to his mother and younger brother, who did nothing to intervene as he grew more and more debilitated. In keeping with a now long-standing pattern, he told only me of his decision to die. My brother and sister were left out of his decision or any opportunity to talk with him about it.

As it had been during my mother's illness, I was intimately drawn into my father's wish to die, while my siblings were left as bystanders. He insisted that I not talk with them. Unfortunately, I honored his request, and looking back I can see now that I felt so estranged from them that it was as though there was no basis for such an intimacy. I could not help them—they were at that time but strangers at the periphery of my life.

I remained horrified and furious with Dad, demanding he take care of himself. He told me to leave him alone—the family's universal solution. I refused. He finally replied, with unforgettable honesty, "You don't have the right to ask that of me. You have not lived my life, and I have had enough of this life." It was a confrontation that would stay with me forever. Even in the last days of his life, he refused to tell me of the war years that still haunted him, but we were able to speak of our lives and losses together in a pained and loving honesty. It was a rare moment of intimacy with my father, a discovery that we did have at least some small capacity to face hard truths together.

My brother and sister did not have the privilege of that kind of conversation with him, and they suffered massively in the face of his death and his determined silence with them. Silences have echoed through our family system. This new silence hid away the secret, the shame and devastation, of our father's passive suicide, a profound abandonment of his children in the earliest stages of their adult lives. Though a hard-working and deeply devoted mother herself, my sister then lived *her* own suffering in silence, *her* history and that of our family lay hidden from her children. My brother has spent most of his life living alone.

Anne Alvarez (2010) examines the psychological and developmental impact of melancholia and mourning in childhood and adolescence. She observes five "particular states of mind" likely to emerge in reaction to unacknowledged and unresolved loss in childhood: paranoia, manic contempt, narcissistic preoccupation, addictive and perverse chuntering, and a state "which has to do with despair, and with those states which go beyond despair into apathy," resulting in an internal object world dominated by "unvalued, as opposed to devalued objects" (p. 4). As I read Alvarez's article, I could see the unconscious impact of the losses and isolation in our family system on each of us—my brother falling into a paranoid state of mind in which any form of attachment was a danger; me into manic contempt in which any form of attachment was a burden and a threat; and my sister into the apathy of an unvalued being, driven only by the desire to avert some of the suffering in her own children's lives. Alvarez comments that children under these circumstances "have had nowhere to put it except on themselves" (p. 13). The Cornell kids did not have a family system capable of helping them do much else than spin off into their own private worlds.

As adults, my brother's and sister's lives were broken and isolated. Debbie, still a teenager, married the first man who showed any interest in her and had four children as quickly as she could, imagining that she would die young like our mother, hoping she could live long enough to get them to adulthood. My sister lived in a violently abusive marriage but was desperate to keep her family together until her kids were grown, believing that she was not worth anything more than the abuse and control her husband heaped upon her. Deb had come, at my invitation, to visit my family in Pittsburgh on a couple of occasions. It was time that we both enjoyed, but our conversations never became personal, and my invitations were never returned to be invited to her home and family. I never met her children. Gradually, we lost touch. I had no contact with my brother, who has never met my children.

In the mid-1990s I received a rare phone call from Deb. She asked directly for my help. She had been beaten by her husband to the point of hospitalization. The hospital moved her directly into a battered women's shelter, where she met for the first time with a psychotherapist. Deb did not see herself as abused; she told the therapist that she deserved her husband's fury. She did not tell the therapist that she made herself the determined target of her husband's rage so as to draw it away from their children. The therapist asked Deb if she would read a couple of articles on trauma and abuse that might help her think about her situation a little a little differently. Deb took the articles in hand, looked up, and said, "My brother Billy wrote one of these articles." I had known nothing about Deb's abuse. The therapist, rather taken aback, suggested she call me.

I helped Deb tentatively separately from her husband. As she was the primary provider in the family, she forced him to leave and took care of her children herself. He repeatedly threatened suicide, begging to return—a scene so typical of households dominated by domestic violence. Deb could not tolerate the thought that her children would lose *their* father to suicide. I doubt she felt she deserved anything better, and she brought him back. She did not tell me of her husband's repeated threats of suicide, she simply let him return to the family. I was forbidden to talk with her unless her husband was on the extension phone. Once again, I withdrew from her anguish.

These were the lives of my siblings that I could not face until confronted by my analyst.

A few years after my divorce, I found my way into a new relationship, this time with a man, also a psychotherapist. He was shocked to learn I had siblings, as his own siblings were a regular part of his life. Deeply versed in Bowen family systems, he was well acquainted with the realities of profound family anxieties, shame, and emotional cutoffs. He suggested an unannounced visit to my sister's home. Although unimaginable to me on my own, we did it. My sister welcomed the two of us into her life with open arms and great relief. Her husband, stunned, did not interfere. Her children, now in their 30s, met Uncle Billy for the first time in their lives. In those few years, Deb and I became very close. This was all the more remarkable to me in that Deb's life experience (she worked in a factory) and worldview were very constrained. She was a blue-collar Republican and was not ashamed of her racist and anti-Semitic views. She had always known me as a married father of three boys, and here I was showing up at her door with a guy. When I asked her about my now being with a man, she said that she was so grateful to him for bringing us together that she simply wanted to get to know the kind of man he was. She said she could see the kind of fathers that he and I were, and she wanted her kids to get to know us. And she could tell I was happy, "and that's enough for me." We began and maintained regular family contact, her husband now on the sidelines.

Then, at 54, Deb was diagnosed with multiple terminal cancers. It was a true blessing that with our reconciliation she did not have to manage her illness and her family's distress by herself. In spite of the odds, she lived two years and remained coherent until a few days before her death.

As she was facing her imminent death, she knew her children needed to know something of her life, her history before she died. But like our father, she could not speak it to them, though they desperately wanted to know her better before they lost her. I was shocked to realize how little, even as adults, they knew about their mother and our family's history. These siblings, three sons and a daughter, had turned to each other to ward off their violent father and to care and be cared for by one another. Deb had been a devoted mother and grandmother, the primary financial provider for the family, while keeping herself the target of her husband's abuse to protect the children. Her kids loved her fiercely, but they did not know her. They could never understand why she chose to stay with their father.

Two weeks before Deb died, now blind and clinging to consciousness, I went to see her alone to talk with her about her funeral. She asked that I speak to her children, for her, about her life. I told her that I had brought a recorder, and we could talk together, and so I could play her own voice to them after she died. She said, "No, I can't." The family legacy of silence was reasserting itself. She wanted to talk to me and for me to then talk to her children for her. She was by this time very ill and blind, so I said to her, "You are fucking blind. I could turn the recorder on, and you'll never know the difference." "If you love me," she replied, "you won't do that. I want to talk to you and you speak for me." I said to her, "You know that's always been my story in the family, Billy will do it." "Well," she said, "Billy is going to do it one more time."

Although it broke her heart, she could not break the silence for her children. That was mine to do as her big brother—a gift to her and her children and grandchildren. At her funeral I spoke of and for my sister, bringing in her own words and voice from our last conversations before she died, what she wanted her children to know but could not speak herself. Her children learned for the first time of their mother's sufferings in her childhood and adult life that had come to shape and limit that life. They had never heard the story of her own mother's tragic illness. They, of course, had had no idea of their grandfather's suicide but could now begin to comprehend why their mother could never leave her husband, their father, for dread of his threatened suicide.

When our brother, Gary, was told that Deb was dying, he replied, "I don't do funerals." Although he could not manage to be with her as she approached death, he did talk with her and came to her funeral. After I spoke, Gary stood and finally gave voice to his own anguish and fury. Here were the generational consequences, the *violence* and *toxicity* of our family's silences and withdrawals, now to be no longer hidden and silent.

Scene Three: Toxic Violence

My second analyst dragged my father into the light of day, focusing a light that was neither kind nor forgiving. Once again there was a sudden, shocking session. I had been dealing with memories of being harassed and terrorized in my early teens by my father's younger brother (whose name I carry as my middle name) on those few occasions when our families were together. There had been a series of turbulent sessions in which I related various experiences, which I had never forgotten, but to which I had never spoken or given any significance—minimizing them, as they had been infrequent. I was apologizing for my father's passive witnessing of his brother's aggressive behavior toward me. My father avoided conflict, and I suspected he had always been afraid of his younger brother. Suddenly, my analyst erupted, threw his notebook and pen across the room and shouted, "*Stop fucking apologizing for your father*. He never did his job!" Once he calmed down, he interpreted my father's withdrawal as a form of violence—a violent, self-serving withdrawal from the work of a father. I did not welcome this news, but I sensed the truth and its implications. Together we examined the ways in which I had internalized my father's crushing shame and self-criticism.

My father was not, in fact, as irresponsible and abandoning as my second analyst had argued, nor as innocent as I preferred to remember him. He was both. My father carried wounds that horribly restricted his own capacity to live, and yet he infused me with a capacity to hungrily seek all that life has to offer. He stepped forward at times in remarkable, thoughtful, and heart-felt ways, doing his damnedest to support my pursuit of a life that he had abandoned for himself. His was not a hostile withdrawal but one he imagined protected us from his inner demons. What I could not see at that time was that while my father's withdrawal was not *hostile*, it was *violent*, and there were aspects of that violence alive in me and lived out through my own isolation and cutting off from care or caring.

I recognized through Apprey's writings that I had indeed accepted and enacted an urgent errand, delivered and fueled by the unmetabolized tragedies of the previous generations. My second analyst had made the violence of this errand impossible to ignore. But I experienced this errand as also profoundly positive, if at times problematic and exhausting. It was, at times, exciting, productive, and a source of admiration from those I admired in return. Apprey attached such adjectives as poisonous, toxic, destructive, aggressive, and violent to his account of these transgenerational errands. Though I could see those adjectives fitting well in the broad, historical, cultural landscapes he inhabited in his writing, I initially could not apply them to my own personal being and history.

Excavating the Debris, Allowing a Future

When Death Leaves Its Traces None of Us Can Remain Unaffected *(Apprey, 2017, p. 17)*

For a number of years, Christopher Bollas (2021) had been coming to Pittsburgh to participate in an ongoing series of independent, clinical seminars at my office called "Keeping Our Work Alive." He had undertaken a series of seminars on character analysis, and one was on the manic character—this one was being delivered over a two-day period. What he said in those two days had a profound impact on my being, much as had my analyst's intervention 15 years earlier.

These are a few of the notes I took during that seminar:

> The manic self to the depressive self, "You are such a drag, a piece of shit."
>
> The manic process raises the mind above its past and created fictive illusions, a virtual self—attempts to create a new past/story/narrative
>
> Panic is avoided by being translated into action. You are panicked about falling into catastrophe, so you are doing everything you can think of to save yourself and the others

In Bollas's words, I could see and feel the violence against myself that lay in the genesis and persistence of my manic ways. Bollas captured both the intrapsychic violence as well as the contempt toward one's own vulnerabilities, against the need or wish to depend. While my first analyst was a rather humble, soft-spoken, classically trained man, my second analyst was rough and tumble, blunt, and outspoken. My first analyst focused on loss and on my conscious and unconscious relations with my mother. My second analyst focused on my father, a man I had protected by leaving him in the shadows until my second analyst confronted me with the violent consequences of my father's withdrawal.

Apprey (1999, 2003) outlines a kind of psychoanalytic archeology, using such terms as "sedimentation," "appropriation," and "intentionality," which have been elaborated upon in prior chapters and which I summarize here in my own words. He starts with the unwanted, split-off debris of a family's history:

1   *Sedimentation*: Herein lies the silenced psychic debris or sediment, the unmetabolized tragedies of the grandparents and parents lives that are banished into silence and secrecy in service of survival. These are the possibly significant events of history and environmental circumstances that live on, unspoken and nearly forgotten, from one generation to the next, as points of disturbed and disturbing significance. These are the grounds from which the ghosts come to haunt and warp the next generation.

2   *Appropriation*: Appropriation is Apprey's term for the process by which an individual begins to concretely live the foundations laid within the sedimentations of the earlier generations, assuming the unconscious *errand* and its expression through which the grievances of history begin to emerge. This errand most often emerges as a transference actualization, usually in the form of negative transferences, which must be received not only as a form of communication between patient and analyst but also as messages/demands from past generations.

3   *Intentionality*: It is here within this realm of appropriation that Apprey seeks to convey the sense of forward intentionality, the unconscious, libidinal forces that seek a future, again enacted in the transference. He suggests, "This new space is saturated with *transference wishes, pleas*, or *demands* made by the subject in order to entertain the possibility of a *reconfiguration that fosters healing under new and favorable conditions*. (2017, p. 36, italics in the original). The analyst is unconsciously called upon to recognize this transferential wish/plea and facilitate its emergence into life. Herein emerges the possibility of a different future, that which Gerson (2017, p. 200) calls "the sustenance for re-creation."

It was my first analyst's pronouncement regarding the place of loss in my psyche and motivation that began to bring voice and meaning to the costs and pain silently endured by my parents. It was through my reading and study with Apprey that I recognized the deeper history of my grandparents and their ancestors. As I tried to look further back to my grandparents, there was so much that I will never come to know. But I could begin to recognize the shadows of dislocation, loss, and cuttings off that left my grandparents without a community and lived history, thus, all too brittle to really live through the fatalities that ruptured the continuities of family histories and fabric. Why it was and whenever it was about that led to my father's ancestors emigration to America is unknown.

Although my maternal grandparents were first-generation immigrants and came to this country with the hopes of so many at that time, these hopes were not realized. It was as though my grandparents and parents were denied any sense of a personal future. Those hopes were then invested in me, my siblings, and cousins. Yet my own generation, numbering ten, was plagued with illnesses, early deaths, addictions, and failed futures. Somehow, I was to be the carrier of the urgent errand, an errand that did in fact, for all of its troubles, propel me into a productive life. Apprey argues, "'Errand' here speaks to the idea that there is someone's intentionality that will come or has come to be made one's own" (2014, p. 17). I was to be a recipient, both willing and unwitting, of that urgency, and that urgency fueled a manic style of life that allowed for neither rest nor the true compassion and companionship of others. I had never expected to live beyond 50, but I have, and in so doing have been able to embrace the love and deep companionship of a partner, friends, and family.

In my analyses, pivotal analytic encounters emerged in the three scenes described previously. Although neither of my analysts was familiar with Apprey's work, each took up these points of crucial therapeutic confrontations and interpretations as opportunities for new, crucial understandings. Each fostered significant changes in my ways of being with myself and others. And each of these crucial analytic scenes has gained new meaning and depth as I have reconsidered them through this lens of transgenerational haunting.

References

Alvarez, A. (2010). Melancholia and mourning in childhood and adolescence: Some reflections on the role of the internal object. In *Enduring Loss: Mourning, Depression, and Narcissism through the Life Cycle*, eds. E. McGinley & A. Varchevker, pp. 3–17. London: Karnac.

Apprey, M. (1999). Reinventing the self in the face of received transgenerational hatred in the African American community. *Journal of Applied Psychoanalytic Studies*, 1(2): 131–143.

Apprey, M. (2003). Repairing history: Reworking transgenerational trauma. In *Hating in the First-Person Plural: Psychoanalytic Essays on Racism, Homophobia, Misogyny, and Terror*, ed. D. Moss, pp. 1–27. New York: Other Press.

Apprey, M. (2006). Difference and the awakening of wounds in intercultural psychoanalysis. *The Psychoanalytic Quarterly*, LXXV(1): 73–93.

Apprey, M. (2014). A pluperfect errand: A turbulent return to beginnings in the transgenerational transmission of destructive aggression. *Free Association: Psychoanalysis and Culture, Media, Groups, Politics*, 66: 16–29.

Apprey, M. (2017). Representing, theorizing and reconfiguring the concept of transgenerational haunting in order to facilitate healing. In *Transgenerational Trauma and the Other*, eds. S. Grand & J. Salberg, pp. 16–37. London: Routledge.

Apprey, M. (2019). "Scripting" inhabitations of unwelcome guests, hosts, and ghosts: Unpacking elements that constitute transgenerational haunting: Interview with William F. Cornell. *Transactional Analysis Journal*, 49(4): 339–351.

Bollas, C. (2021). *Three Characters: Narcissist, Borderline, Manic Depressive*. Oxfordshire: Phoenix Publishing House.

Gerson, S. (2017). Afterword. In *Ghosts in the Consulting Room: Echoes of Trauma in Psychoanalysis*, eds. A. Harris, M. Kalb & S. Klebanoff, pp. 199–203. London: Routledge.

Schwab, G. (2010). *Haunting Legacies: Violent Histories and Transgenerational Trauma*. New York: Columbia University Press.

Afterword

Temporality and Apprey's Hauntology for Psychoanalysis

Michael Uebel

In this book, Apprey, a pioneer in the study of psychic phenomena express-ing transgenerational transmissions of aggressivity, brilliantly shows the implications of such transmissibility for psychoanalytic theory and therapy. Taking Freud's instinct theory and radically reworking it into an object relations theory that can better account for the temporality of psychic messaging, Apprey offers various strategies for conceptualizing how humans enact and make sense of history. Yet, of Apprey's *drama-tis personae*, Freud is not the central character. Nor are the philoso-phers Husserl, Heidegger, Merleau-Ponty, Jean-Luc Marion, Claude Romano, et alia—all of whom Apprey mobilizes with total perspicacity. The main figure turns out to be the poet W.H. Auden, whose celebrated 1937 poem "On This Island" with its line juxtaposing the urgent and the voluntary in a ship's errand prompted Apprey to think through the seeming contradictions embedded in the poetic phrase: Under what con-ditions are errands *voluntary*? And, further, if errands are truly *urgent*, then what room is left for choice, the spontaneous? Auden's "errands" would orient Apprey, like the diverging ships in the poem, sending him on a multiplex psychoanalytic errand of his own. Apprey embarked on nothing less than on a career-defining mission to formulate how subjects may become doubly trapped and imperiled by the infused toxicity of ancestral legacies of aggression and by the often self-destructive choices they make.

Without privileging one disciplinary approach over others, Apprey allows the insights offered by philosophy, psychology, and fictional media (especially film) to fluidly inform his readings of the psyche's hidden sedi-mentations of history and their toxic reanimations. Apprey the psychoana-lyst listens to these otherwise silent layers, noting when they come to life

DOI: 10.4324/9781003389026-16

and observing how they are ultimately refashioned to serve contemporary functions. This rich and generous book teaches others how to do the same. It encourages us never to believe that understanding human behavior, cognition, and affect can occur in isolation from deep appreciation of the manifold ways they have been historically conditioned. Apprey's brilliant deployment of semiology, phenomenology, and Freudian metapsychology yields a number of templates and conceptual lenses for grasping the tensions inhering in the psychic space between unconsciously absorbed toxic forces from the external world and the unconsciously appropriated toxic intrusions he calls internal "dreams" of "urgent voluntary errands."

The book's central theme, as I see it, is temporality. For all the elucidations of gaps, borders, sedimentations, aporias, dislocations, wanderings, lines, and sutures—some of Apprey's recurring tropes—the spatial imagery never manages to obscure the significance of the flow of time and the transport of history. Temporality, it turns out, is quite spatial, and this is as it should be. In Apprey's account, it flows backwards and forwards. We live in space and time, and any understanding of what it means to move forward—say, in an analysis or life—confronts us with openness, which we usually comprehend spatially. The open world becomes the salvific aspect of analysis. And while there may be some who still believe Freudianism and pessimism coincide, despite pessimism's various undoings in different brands of ego psychology from Alfred Adler to Erik Erikson, the psychoanalytic project has always, even at times strangely, been amenable to futurity. This openness to the future in Freud is expressed, among other places, in the idea that analysis is *unendliche* (interminable). Following Freud's lessons in "Analysis Terminable and Interminable" (1937a) and "Constructions in Analysis" (1937b), we may conclude that all that analysis can do is "decide" its own provisional end. It can never celebrate the discovery of a truth rescued from oblivion. Analysis must therefore content itself with historicizing not the truth but the subject's conviction of the truth and, in this way, working through all the contradictions such conviction produces. Never reaching a foundation where, as Freud (1914) writes in "On Narcissism," "everything rests" (p. 77), the analytic construction enjoys no special privilege as any sort of totalizing critique.

I suspect Apprey might agree with this, or so this is the impression I get from the book when he states (and demonstrates) that what so deeply interests him is the sense of history that is translated from the events of history.

The Freudian object, like the Nietzschean one, is after all the "power of truth," wherein truth has meaning precisely as an operation whose immunity to criticism extends even to the point where it is said to contradict reality. Accordingly, we are bound by the terms of our reality sense: "We cannot escape this world," Freud insists in *Civilization and Its Discontents* (1930); "we are always within it" (p. 65).[1] Being within, as Freud's poetic essay "On Transience" (1916) makes clear, is preeminently a condition of temporality, an alienated relation to the cruelty and finitude of natural life. In the end, there is no retreat "outside" or "beyond" this world, with even the mysterious unconscious itself an impossible refuge for some discoverable truth about the self. The unconscious is, after all, *unheimlich* (un-homely, a-topic) and atemporal, with its multiplicity of desires shattering every illusion of linear progress toward truth.[2] Franco Rella, in *Myth of the Other*, sums it up like this, in terms I must admit Apprey might not endorse: "Outside of this reality there exists no lost homeland, no possibility of escape from alienation—the Freudian *Unheimliche*—from this plurality, from this network of contradictions that characterize and 'perturb' our desire" (p. 30).

Apprey offers lines of escape, as his case studies of individuals and groups reveals. He writes convincingly about psychological liberation, the freedom to return to the self that results when an analysand resubjectivizes her own exit strategy from ghostly immurement, beginning a gradual process of psychic emancipation. The archaic mandate to die and the experiential structures entombing and decaying the self are abandoned in favor of growth, of life. A toxic errand can be transformed into a salutary one by attending to and naming historical traumas and generating the willingness to change. Freedom can be found even if everything is not explicated, despite it not all being analyzed away. Indeed, Freudian analysis teaches us that, in the absence of a substitute for our "civilization's discontent," there is left only the possibility of critically describing *our own* historical and cultural discontent. The labor of analytic description is thus by its nature contingent, incomplete, and, because it occurs within the time of crisis and unhappiness, risky. Freud saw the necessary incompleteness of critical description, what he termed *die Mängel unserer Beschreibung* (*Jenseits des Lustprinzips*, p. 65) as the only construction or interpretation of which we can be sure. The time of analysis, it seems, is necessarily partial or fragmentary, as Freud's (1905) experience of the curtailed analysis of Dora, his first great case study, dramatizes.[3]

Apprey points us then toward something very important: by naming the gap, the phantom incompleteness inhering in psychic life, where the secrets introjected by anterior or ancestral objects transmit destructive aggression, an escape path is illumined, like an aircraft's emergency lighting system. I was pleased in this regard to see that apparently Apprey is as fond of the ideas of Nicolas Abraham (1988) as I am, specifically his notion that phantoms per se do not really haunt; the revenants and demons who unsettle history constitute suppressed experiences of the other, objectifications of "the gaps left within us by the secrets of others" (p. 75). In a sense, we silently carry our unsuccessful mournings related to all the toxicity left in need of expression. So, what returns to haunt is the "tomb of the other" which otherwise would have remained buried, suppressed as part of the other's reality. And so, here Apprey comes close to Freud's (1909) observation that, in analysis, "a thing which has not been understood inevitably reappears like an unlaid ghost, it cannot rest until the mystery has been solved and the spell broken" (p. 122).

One of the metapsychological points to grapple with here is that, for Freud (1923), the unconscious knows nothing of time, is timeless, and hence "no unconscious correlate can be found" for death (p. 58). Death, the finality of time, leaves no traces in the unconscious for Freud, whereas for Lacan (2006a), the death of things is the very predicate for claiming that one is alive. Symbolization, the putting of reality into language, strips things of their "thing-ness" and at the same time guarantees the continuity of desire: "the symbol first manifests itself as the killing of the thing, and this death results in the endless perpetuation of the subject's desire" ("Function and Field of Speech in Language," p. 262). Lacan's account of the emergence of the symbolic order through the death of the thing is important to both his theory of temporality and his theory of intersubjectivity, for it is precisely when things assume a relation to other things that they can be said to have duration in time. Objects have a temporal duration that is bestowed upon them when two or more subjects together establish a symbolic world, and they do this through naming: "the name is the time of the object" (*The Seminar of Jacques Lacan, Book 2*, p. 169).

Apprey's declaration that "any account of human nature that fails to take serious account of history and culture will be inadequate" brings before us the necessity and value of acts of naming. As Lacan's (2006a) "Logical Time" essay shows, the rules of the game are structured around the act of naming. The "game" that Lacan describes—there are three prisoners and five discs (three white and two black), one of which is placed on each inmate's back by a warden who announces that the first one who can identify his own color and do so according to "logical and not simply probabilistic grounds" (p. 161) wins his freedom—is more than mere sophistry. It is a matter of the assertion of identity, where the fundamental question posed is: How do I name myself, declare my subjectivity, as in "I am . . . "? Lacan's answer was that it could be done with a degree of certainty only if the dialectical categories of time (life/death, memory/oblivion, past/future) were reorganized around waiting/concluding. In its most basic formulation, this new dialectical relation of hesitation and conclusion provides the source of what Lacan calls "subjective logic," in other words, a logic based in a time whose intersubjective condition becomes an allegory for the psychoanalytic process, the time of analysis. In the game-theory model of the three prisoners, waiting assumes a logical function whereby one arrives at a solution to the question of subjectivity through a process of decision-making in relation to one's fellow human beings. Subjective time is thus filled with "the time for understanding"—in Lacan's schema, the logical period between the "the instant of the gaze" and "the moment to conclude"—a time not without its obsessional and narcissistic symptomatology[4] and one that, over the course of an analysis, will be annulled in favor of moments of concluding. This period is the one in which the subject assumes his history, and, together with the moment of concluding, it constitutes the Freudian *durcharbeiten* (working-through).

I detect in Apprey's work a convergence with Lacan's (2006b) insight that "analysis can have as its goal only . . . the subject's realization of his history in its relation to a future" ("Function and Field of Speech in Language," p. 249). The assumption, by the subject, of the past and the future takes place through the mode of interlocution—"speech addressed to the other"—where the effect of psychoanalytic anamnesis is "to reorder past contingencies by conferring on them the sense of necessities to come" (ibid., p. 213). The analyst's neutrality, which Lacan (1983) says "takes its true meaning from the position of the pure dialectician," opens up the possibility for the subject's "becoming," a process involving the ongoing projection of history into discourse (p. 72). This projection of the past into language is not the mere articulation of what one has been; rather, it is an enunciation of what one will have been. The temporal structure of the subject may be specified, following Heidegger's *Being and Time*, as "futural" or, defined in terms of tense, as that of the future anterior.[5] Psychoanalysis views the past history of the subject in terms of a time that can never be fully remembered because it can never be said to have fully taken place. The subject is inscribed within the inclusive temporality of the "will-always-already-have-been" (*Immerschongewesen-sein-wird*), a time that is always yet to come, in Heidegger's formula, a "being towards" (*Sein zu*). The opacity of this terminology aside, what this means for the subject of the unconscious is that it cannot grasp its history because certain elements of the past are always to be anticipated belatedly.

We can understand then the future past of the subject as at the same time a mode of existence and a commentary on the possibility of (doing or making sense of) history: "History is not the past. History is not the past in so far as it is historicized in the present—historicized in the present because it was lived in the past" (Lacan, *The Seminar of Jacques Lacan, Book 1*, p. 12).[6] History involves an identification with what one will have been, as for example when Freud writes to Wilhelm Fliess in 1900 to express his desire that "someday one will read on a marble tablet on this house: 'Here, on July 24, 1895,/the secret of the dream/revealed itself to Dr. Sgm. Freud'" (Masson, 1985, p. 417). This expression of a wish or an ideal ego reads, indeed works, backward from a time in the future when Freud's discovery will have been publicly acclaimed. The retroactive (*nachträglich*) temporal structure of the fantasy here amounts not to a memorializing of the (future) past but to a manipulation of it, along with the present, in relation to the future. To put this another way, the past momentarily suspends the present so that the future becomes an open question, a possibility. The present is in effect left for another time. In the structure of fantasy, wish fulfillment, and even utopia, where among the three temporal orders, it is the past that, from the perspective of psychoanalysis, is most fluid, meaning is only created ex post facto, never instantaneously.[7] The subject, always either about to arrive (i.e., on the verge of arriving) or will have already arrived, thus remains in a rhythm of abeyance or suspense. The former temporal mode is at work in Fourier and de Sade and the latter in Marx and Thoreau.

For Apprey, the subject on the verge of arriving is one who must negotiate a return involving the coincidence of the present and the past unconscious, in order to carry out an errand that is both one's own and the Other's. Yet the future must remain open. This is where I think Apprey recrafts Derrida's (1994) hauntology, where the presence of the ghost poses the problem of the event as both originary and repeating. Here's what I mean: selfhood undergoes constant revision and disruption when new relations to some originary event are formed. In serial identities formation, as in the Freudian analysis of neurosis, the question whether the originary event really "came before" (as, say, part of an infantile past) or is really the product of subsequent fantasy is of secondary importance. What matters is the retroactive force that an encounter with otherness exerts on the present subject. Coming after the subject, the other addresses it as its cause, and in so doing throws the subject radically into question:

> The desire of the Other puts me in question [*me met en cause*], it interrogates me at the very root of my own desire as *a*, as cause of this desire and not as object. And because this is what the Other targets, in a temporal relation of antecedence, I can do nothing to break this hold, except to engage with it.
>
> (Lacan, 2014, p. 153)

This temporal dimension is equated to anxiety, the very reason so many patients come to us seeking help.

To reframe Freud, as Apprey does, helps us, he states, be "aware that we often think we are experientially going somewhere only to realize that we have already been there. Or, we think we have a project only to realize that we have already been sent." Remarkably, Freud (1920), in a brief commentary on the "Kantian theorem" that time is a "necessary form of thought" (p. 28), suggests that the claim about the unconscious as timeless is itself a theorem about time strictly from the perspective of consciousness. Freud claims that one can only understand the "negative characteristics" of the unconscious—that is, its temporal disorder and resistance to change by time—by comparing unconscious mental processes with conscious ones. From such a comparison, the following conclusion, which Freud (1920) admits "must sound very obscure," might be drawn:

> our abstract idea of time seems to be wholly derived from the method of working of the [perceptual-conscious system] . . . and to correspond to a perception on its own part of that method of working. This mode of functioning may perhaps constitute another way of providing a shield against stimuli.
>
> (p. 28)[8]

The perceptual system, oscillating between the defense against and reception of stimuli, or, as we might rephrase it, fluctuating between pleasure and unpleasure, is responsible for our time sense.[9] As Freud (1925) put it in "A Note on the Mystic Writing-Pad," "the periodic non-excitability of the perceptual system," its "discontinuous method of functioning . . . lies at the bottom of the origin of the concept of time" (p. 231). It is the dialectical nature of perception, involving moments of unreceptivity or repose, rather than simply a self-examining consciousness (as for Kant) or continuous feeling and thinking (as for Bergson), whose logic of interruptions, according to Lacan (2006a), "reveal[s] itself at each moment as the subjective unfolding of a temporal instance" ("Logical Time," p. 166).

This unfolding of the temporal instant produces the possibility for seeing things anew, for tracing the rhythms and movements of (internal and external) objects or images that relentlessly confront us with their sheer inevitability and finality. In this important sense, as Bachelard (1990) put it, "time must therefore be taught" (p. 49). The challenges of teaching time are, however, rarely met, indeed sometimes wholly unacknowledged, yet the present book meets and exceeds those challenges. Apprey, a brilliant teacher and healer of time, shows how the dialectic of movement and finality, beginnings and endings, deferments and willed actions all play out across personal histories in ways that necessitate progressive and retrogressive evaluations on the part of the analyst.

Notes

1 Freud was fond of this quotation from Christian Dietrich Grabbe's edgy historical drama *Hannibal* [1835]; he cites it, for example, in a letter to Lou Andreas-Salomé, dated 30 July 1915: *Sigmund Freud and Lou Andreas-Salomé: Letters*, ed. E. Pfeiffer; trans. William and E. Robson-Scott (New York: W.W. Norton, 1985), p. 32.

2 Rella summarizes: "Outside of this reality there exists no lost homeland, no possibility of escape from alienation—the Freudian *Unheimliche*—from this plurality, from this network of contradictions that characterize and 'perturb' our desire": *Myth of the Other*, p. 30. "Atopy" is Rella's neologism for approximating the Freudian *Unheimliche*, thereby underscoring its alienating affectivity—the lack of home or place, being away from one's homeland. For the development of the term, see Rella, F. (1987). *Limina*. Milan: Feltrinelli.

3 A fine discussion of this case as one that "oscillates endlessly between [Freud's] desire for complete insight or knowledge and an unconscious realization (or fear) of the fragmentary, deferring status of knowledge itself " is offered by

Moi, T. (1985). Representation of patriarchy: Sexuality and epistemology in Freud's Dora. In *In Dora's Case: Freud—Hysteria—Feminism*, eds. C. Bernheimer & C. Kahane, pp. 181–199. New York: Columbia University Press; see especially pp. 184–187.

4 See Samuels, R. (1990). Logical time and jouissance. *Newsletter of the Freudian Field*, 4: 69–77; esp. 71–72.

5 The "future anterior" is also known as the "future perfect," a particularly equivocal tense in French, and one exploited by Lacan in his writings. The "futural" belongs to philosophy: "By the term 'futural,'" Heidegger writes, "we do not here have in view a 'now' which has *not yet* become 'actual' and which sometime *will be* for the first time. We have in view the coming [*Kunft*] in which Dasein, in its own most potentiality-for-Being, comes toward itself." As Heidegger goes on to specify it in the next paragraph, he has in mind a future that constitutes "what will-have-been": "Only so far as it is futural can Dasein be authentically as having been. The character of 'having been' arises, in a certain way, from the future": Heidegger, M. (1962). *Being and Time*. Translated by J. Macquarrie & E. Robinson. New York: Harper Collins, p. 373.

6 Compare with Sartre: "I am not my past. I am not my past because I was my past": Sartre, J.-P. (1976). *L'etre et le néant: essai d'ontologie phénoménologique*. 1943; repr. Paris: Gallimard, p. 154.

7 Recall Freud's early "extreme" position on memories: "It may indeed be questioned whether we have any memories at all from our childhood: memories relating to our childhood may be all that we possess": Screen memories. In *Standard Edition*, Volume 3, pp. 322 [303–322]. If all memories are screen memories, then it is senseless to look behind such screens to some "original, primal" trace. Derrida's critique of truth as a disclosing is an important commentary on this: "Le facteur de la vérité," in Derrida, J. (1987). *The Post Card: From Socrates to Freud and Beyond*. Translated by A. Bass. Chicago: University of Chicago Press, pp. 413–496.

8 The radical theoretical extension of this "obscure" statement—that conscious time is itself a repudiation of or stimulus barrier to unconscious time, with its tension-raising *eros* and narcissism—is explored by Bass, A. (2000). *Difference and Disavowal: The Trauma of Eros*. Stanford: Stanford University Press, pp. 83–86 and 237.

9 Recent psychoanalytic theory emphasizes this correlation of temporality and affectivity where the notion of time is acquired by the infant as she experiences objects as alternately fulfilling of needs or satisfying and frustrating. The affective dimensions of adult psychopathology then become explicable in terms of time. For example, depression is associated with a pathological relation to the past and anxiety with one to the future. And, most importantly for our purposes, timelessness is theorized, as in the previous Freud quotation, as a defensive retreat from an unpleasurable awareness of time or history. For theory on temporality and mind after Freud, see Arlow, J. (1989). Time as emotion. In *Time and Mind: Interdisciplinary Issues*, ed. J. T. Fraser, pp. 85–97. Madison, CT: International Universities Press, and Hartocollis, P. (1983). *Time and Timelessness, or The Varieties of Temporal Experience*. New York: International Universities Press.

References

Abraham, N. (1988). Notes on the phantom: A complement to Freud's metapsychology (Trans. Nicholas Rand). In *The Trial(s) of Psychoanalysis*, ed. F. Meltzer, pp. 75–80. Chicago: University of Chicago Press.

Bachelard, G. (1990). *The Dialectic of Duration*. Translated by M. McAllester Jones. Manchester: Clinamen Press.

Derrida, J. (1994). *Specters of Marx: The State of the Debt, the Work of Mourning, and the New International*. Translated by P. Kamuf. New York: Routledge.

Freud, S. (1905). Fragment of an analysis of a case of hysteria. In *Standard Edition*, Volume 7, pp. 3–122. London: Hogarth Press.

Freud, S. (1909). Analysis of phobia in a five-year-old boy. In *Standard Edition*, Volume 10, pp. 5–149. London: Hogarth Press.

Freud, S. (1914). On narcissism: An introduction. In *Standard Edition*, Volume 14, pp. 73–102. London: Hogarth Press.

Freud, S. (1916). On transience. In *Standard Edition*, Volume 14, pp. 305–307. London: Hogarth Press.

Freud, S. (1920). Beyond the pleasure principle. In *Standard Edition*, Volume 18, pp. 7–64. London: Hogarth Press.

Freud, S. (1923). The ego and the id. In *Standard Edition*, Volume 19, pp. 12–66. London: Hogarth Press.

Freud, S. (1925). A note on the mystic writing-pad. In *Standard Edition*, Volume 19, pp. 227–232. London: Hogarth Press.

Freud, S. (1930). Civilization and its discontents. In *Standard Edition*, Volume 21, pp. 64–145. London: Hogarth Press.

Freud, S. (1937a). Analysis terminable and interminable. In *Standard Edition*, Volume 23, pp. 216–253. London: Hogarth Press.

Freud, S. (1937b). Constructions in analysis. In *Standard Edition*, Volume 23, pp. 257–269. London: Hogarth Press.

Freud, S. (1940). *Jenseits des Lustprinzips*, Volume 13 of Gesammelte Werke, 17 vols., pp. 3–69. Frankfurt am Main: S. Fischer Verlag.

Lacan, J. (1983). Intervention on transference (Trans. Jacqueline Rose). In *Feminine Sexuality: Jacques Lacan and the École Freudienne*, eds. J. Mitchell & J. Rose, pp. 61–73. New York: W.W. Norton.

Lacan, J. (1988). *The Seminar of Jacques Lacan, Book 2: The Ego in Freud's Theory and in the Technique of Psychoanalysis, 1954–1955*. Edited by J.-A. Miller; Translated by S. Tomaselli. New York: W.W. Norton.

Lacan, J. (1991). *The Seminar of Jacques Lacan, Book 1: Freud's Papers on Technique, 1953–1954*. Edited by J.-A. Miller; Translated by J. Forrester. New York: W.W. Norton.

Lacan, J. (2006a). Logical time and the assertion of anticipated certainty: A new sophism. In *Ecrits: The First Complete Edition in English*, trans. B. Fink, pp. 161–175. New York: W.W. Norton.

Lacan, J. (2006b). The function and field of speech and language in psychoanalysis. In *Ecrits: The First Complete Edition in English*, ed. J. Lacan; trans. B. Fink, pp. 197–268. New York: W.W. Norton.

Lacan, J. (2014). *Anxiety: The Seminar of Jacques Lacan, Book X*. Edited by J.-A. Miller; Translated by A. R. Price. Malden, MA: Polity Press.

Masson, J. M. (Ed.). (1985). *The Complete Letters of Sigmund Freud to Wilhelm Fliess, 1887–1904*. Cambridge, MA: Harvard University Press.

Rella, F. (1994). *The Myth of the Other: Lacan, Deleuze, Foucault, Bataille*. Translated by N. Moe. Washington, DC: Maisonneuve Press.

Index

For Product Safety Concerns and Information please contact our EU
representative GPSR@taylorandfrancis.com
Taylor & Francis Verlag GmbH, Kaufingerstraße 24, 80331 München, Germany

9 7 8 1 0 3 2 4 8 4 3 0 3